What they're saying about Dr. Patrick Nuzzo and *Naprapathy, Manual Medicine for the 21st Century*:

I have enjoyed the distinct honor of knowing Dr. Patrick Nuzzo for more than three decades, and his commitment to improving the lives of his patients, his unbelievable diligence as a well-respected healthcare professional and his passion for his chosen field of expertise, Naprapathy, shows itself on every page of this informative book.

As the head trainer for a professional sports franchise, I see first-hand how connective tissue chronic pain can drastically impact performance and even shorten careers.

In *Naprapathy, Manual Medicine for The 21st Century*, Dr. Nuzzo shows the lay reader how this old-yet-new field of medicine directly addresses the epidemic of chronic pain incidents in the country, might reverse the opioid addiction curse faced by many Americans and improves the overall quality of life for so many people, whether elite athletes competing on the highest levels or anyone else hoping to return to a normal quality of life.

Dr. Nuzzo's Naprapathy has something for everyone interested in just feeling better.

-- Herm Schneider
Head Trainer, Chicago White Sox

I have been blessed to have joined Dr. Nuzzo and Dr. LaVista on their journey to reform healthcare for the better at Southwest University of Naprapathic Medicine. They have opened my eyes to a branch of medicine that is desperately needed in an era of opioid addiction.

As a doctor of chiropractic medicine and the director of sports medicine for the world renowned Jacksonwink MMA Academy, I became aware that there was a large gap in musculoskeletal care related to connective tissue treatment and manual therapy. Naprapathic Medicine safely and effectively fills that gap. Learning under Dr. Nuzzo has drastically improved my outcomes as a clinician, and has allowed multiple MMA world champions to continue their career long after traditional doctors had told them they were finished.

Naprapathic Medicine improves outcomes, decreases reliance on unnecessary drugs and surgery, and dramatically reduces overall healthcare costs through conservative manual medicine.

This book is an outstanding resource for the lay person and clinician alike to understand the history, principals, and mission of a profession that is destined to help turn around our healthcare crisis. Dr. Nuzzo combines his vast knowledge of physiology, his extensive clinical expertise, and his compassion and relate-ability in patient care to give us the most complete textbook on Naprapathy in existence.

– Dr. Beau Hightower, D.N., D.C.
Director, Jacksonwink MMA Academy

Naprapathy

Manual Medicine
for
The 21st Century

By Dr. Patrick Nuzzo, D.N.
And Dr. Kirsten LaVista, D.N.

Cover Model: Lais DeLeon
www.laisdeleon.com

Photography by Shayla Edenfield Photography
http://www.shaylaedenfieldphotography.com

Lais DeLeon
http://laisdeleonfitness.com/

Southwest University of Naprapathic Medicine
2006 Butolph Road, Suite A
Santa Fe, New Mexico 87505

ISBN: 978-0-578-40223-9

DEDICATION

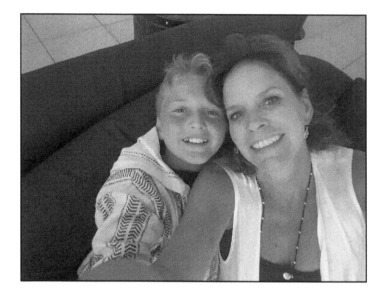

To Kirsten, who's partnership, loyalty, integrity and
persistence has made it all possible – this book,
Naprapathic Medicine of New Mexico,
the Southwest University of Naprapathic Medicine,
our sweet, beautiful son and our blessed journey.
I thank you with all my heart and hands.

Patrick

CONTENTS

ACKNOWLEDGMENTS

We owe a debt of gratitude to many people who gave their assistance for this book, including our patients at Naprapathic Medicine of New Mexico, especially those who agreed to share their personal stories on these pages; the students of the Southwest University of Naprapathic Medicine; my colleagues; those brilliant teachers and practitioners we learned from; the State of New Mexico for its embrace of Naprapathy and encouragement to create SUNM; and so many others who influenced and participated in creating this story of Naprapathic Manual Medicine. We hope all their kindness and assistance will be rewarded with unending health and happiness.

Dr. Patrick Nuzzo, D.N.
Dr. Kirsten LaVista, D.N.

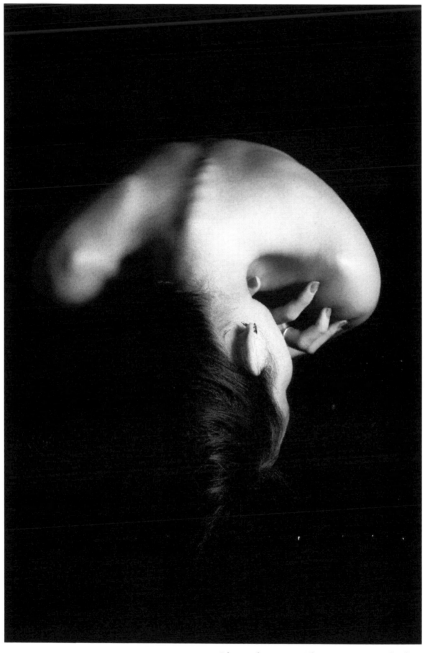

Photo by Jairo Alzate on Unsplash

INTRODUCTION

NAPRAPATHY – HANDS-ON HELP FOR MUSCULOSKELETAL MISERY

In the old country – Bohemia then, the Czech Republic today – they called it "Napravit." It was, then as now, a method of manual medicine used to treat the aches, strains, and injuries that we all so easily acquire in our daily lives. Farmers and laborers in the mostly rural, agrarian countryside of Central Europe sought such remedies to help them to accomplish their daily tasks, when physical ailments otherwise threatened to leave them incapacitated and unable to work or care for their families.

The origins of Naprapathic treatment are rooted in the urgency they had to get better, fast, to go about their daily lives. During the late 19th century, when millions of Europeans migrated to America, often with little more than the clothes on their backs, they brought along the knowledge that helped them survive the tough life they had in their home countries, and would help them master the tough life they faced in the New World. They knew empirically that a system of manual manipulation would help the bad backs, sciatica episodes, nerve pain, muscle weakness and other infirmities that stood between them and the absolute need to get up the next morning and make a living.

Fast forward to today and things are not much different. Certainly, our jobs are more "modern," assisted by new methods and machines, done more in

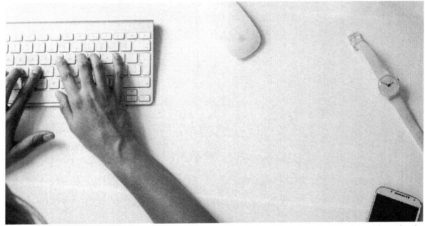

Photo by Damien Zaleski on Unsplash

offices and commercial buildings than in fields and farms and early factories. But our human bodies, evolving not quite as fast as our technology, are still prone to stress and injury from the way we live our lives. In fact, with all the inventions of the past 150 years – from electric lights, to automobiles and airplanes, to laptops and iPads – we have also invented new ways to make ourselves physically miserable.

Indeed, our human precursors evolved the opposable thumb as long as 5 million years ago, but it has taken us only about five decades to disable that long history of evolution with carpal tunnel syndrome,

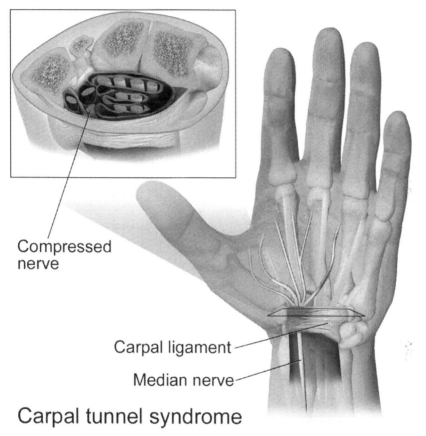

Compressed nerve

Carpal ligament

Median nerve

Carpal tunnel syndrome

Blausen.com staff (2014).
"Medical gallery of Blausen Medical 2014".
WikiJournal of Medicine 1 (2).
DOI:10.15347/wjm/2014.010. ISSN 2002-4436.

the "repetitive strain injury" that causes pain, numbness and immobility in the thumb and other fingers, along with a multitude of other ailments.

That's progress for you. And it's just one example of the new problems we inflict on ourselves with our contemporary lifestyles. If you haven't heard of "text neck," you will.

* * * * *

It was an Iowa-trained practitioner who created the profession that today is Naprapathy (nuh-PRAH-path-y), a profession whose specialty it is to treat exactly

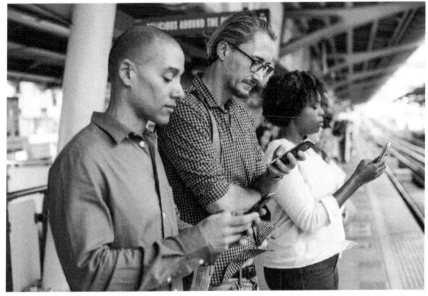

Photo by Rawpixel on Unsplash

those problems.   Dr. Oakley Smith, who learned chiropractic medicine in the early 20th century at the hands of its primary American promulgator, D.D. Palmer, soon realized that what he had studied at Palmer's School of Cure in Davenport, Iowa, was not really what he was observing in his practice. The way he saw physical ailments manifesting led him beyond the mere question of spinal misalignment (called "subluxation") to what he believed was the cause of misalignment in the first place. Dr. Smith's theory put the root of the problem in the soft tissues rather than the bones.   Stresses and strains that affected the myriad of connective tissues in our bodies – the tendons, ligaments, cartilage and fascia that literally keep us from falling apart all over the sidewalk – pulled the vertebrae out of place and created all kinds of problems.

As a good scientist, Dr. Smith sought proof for his theory, and found it in the pathology lab looking at connective tissue under the microscope. What he saw were adhesions affecting the nerves after they emerged from the spine, cumulative trauma that constricted nerve impulses and instead caused pain, muscle tension, numbness, partial paralysis and other infirmities that kept patients from their activities. These strictures also affected the blood and lymph vessels that form bundles with the nerves, bringing oxygen and nourishment, as well as carrying away metabolic waste products from our muscles and organs.

Dr. Smith realized that by freeing up the connective tissue – in particular the fascia that surrounds every organ, separates all of our 650-plus muscles from other muscles and tissue, and supports our bodies' structure – he could relieve pain and dysfunction.

He was also aware of the manual manipulations used by Central European immigrants to help their fellows, and saw that they were in fact treating exactly the syndrome he had seen in the lab. Dr. Smith studied their methods intensely, even traveling to Bohemia for an extended term to learn at the source. With what he found and codified, he sought to "modernize" chiropractic, but indeed founded a new branch of manual medicine entirely:

Naprapathy – the subject of this book.

* * * * *

The intervening century-plus since Oakley Smith seems sometimes to have been a steady string of medical miracles – new diagnostics, new procedures, new therapies, and new pharmaceuticals – and certainly many of the developments and discoveries have lengthened and improved our lives, but some of the "advancements" have proven to be anything but.

National Institutes of Health
National Center for Complementary and Integrative Health

Pain in the U.S.

 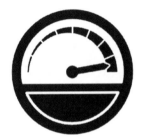

25.3 million
**American adults
suffer from daily pain**

23.4 million
**American adults
report a lot of pain**

Nahin RL. Estimates of Pain Prevalence and Severity in Adults. United States, 2012.
Journal of Pain (2015); doi: 10.1016/j.jpain.2015.05.002.

 National Center for
Complementary and
Integrative Health

nccih.nih.gov/health/pain

The opioid crisis of the early 21st century is a sad and discouraging example. Some 72 percent of those with back pain will attempt to treat it with drugs, and the results have often been addiction and the societal woes we see on the evening news.

Yet, the aches and pains, the disabilities and the dysfunctions, continue pretty much unabated. According to studies from the University of North Carolina and other researchers, as many as 80 percent of Americans at some point in their lives will suffer from chronic back pain.

However, there are effective and benign alternatives, treatments that are proven to relieve our pain and infirmities, that are complementary to other forms of medical treatment – physical therapy, as an example, which focuses on exercises to strengthen muscles where weakness or injury has caused pain and disability. Unlike PT, in which the therapist in most cases follows a prescription in determining care for a patient, Naprapathy combines both diagnosis and treatment. A Doctor of Naprapathy (DN) looks at signs, symptoms and patient history to determine the right course to follow, and then provides the treatment.

It is a tenet of Naprapathy that the initial signs of improvement – e.g., relief from pain, restoration of free movement – are to be expected after one or perhaps two, treatments, unlike the 8-12 that can often be required with medical doctor-prescribed PT, and the uncertain (though admittedly soothing) effects from a course of massage therapy or other manual treatments. Naprapathy, going back to its roots, exists to get people back to their daily activities quickly and efficiently. If, after a third treatment, improvement is not apparent to the patient or practitioner, a Naprapathic Physician will likely refer you to an MD to evaluate whether yours is a condition that needs treatment beyond the scope of Naprapathic practice. Naprapathy does not make the claims of some other disciplines that it can treat or cure conditions that cannot be seen and felt by the Naprapathic Physician.

* * * * *

In the pages that follow, readers will learn many things about their bodies they have probably never given thought to. But with a little reflection the logic will quickly become apparent, and the Naprapathic modality of treatment understood as an effective, fast, non-invasive and non-injurious way to improve their lives.

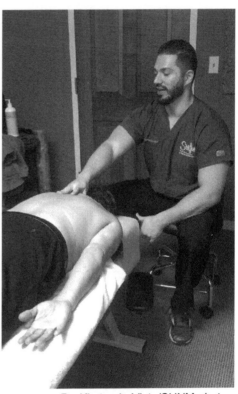

Dr. Kirsten LaVista/SUNM photo

Muskuloskeletal pain is more than an epidemic in this country. Along with the billions of dollars it costs our society in disability and lost productivity, it is the cause of other catastrophic health crises – in particular rampant addiction to opioid drugs. It does not have to be that way. Naprapathy, though little known, has great potential to help millions of people. The chapters of this book will arm sufferers with the knowledge of an old, yet new, way to get better and live the lives they desire – and deserve – to enjoy.

CHAPTER ONE

WHAT IS NAPRAPATHY?

I t is a daily refrain in professional medical offices:

"I need to go back to work."

"I want to be able to pick up my kids."

"I can't sleep because of the pain."

"I just want to feel like my old self again."

Patients are looking for help to get through their daily lives productively and successfully, but their bodies don't always cooperate. Yes, human beings have a super computer in their heads, a cardiovascular engine that keeps every organ and muscle running non-stop for decades, and a nutrition processing plant in their bellies that fuels the fires and keeps us on the go.

On the musculoskeletal side, the human body is an amazing biomechanical machine that is constantly working – even when standing still or sitting on the couch your muscles tense and relax continually to keep you upright. But like all machines that get used a lot, from your car to your lawnmower to the hard drive in your computer, things sometimes get out of sorts and need repairs.

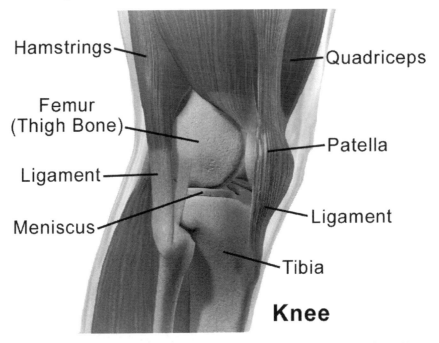

Hamstrings

Quadriceps

Femur
(Thigh Bone)

Patella

Ligament

Ligament

Meniscus

Tibia

Knee

Hard and soft tissue of the knee joint, including the meniscus or cartilage that cushions the bones, and the ligaments.

Blausen.com staff (2014). "Medical gallery of Blausen Medical 2014". WikiJournal of Medicine 1 (2). DOI:10.15347/wjm/2014.010. ISSN 2002-4436.

Form and function are the key starting points in any design – whether it's your home, your iPhone or your physical shape. In the human body, form starts with the skeleton, those 206 bones (in an adult, another hundred in a newborn baby) that define us as an upright, bipedal, opposable-thumbed member of the animal kingdom with a brain pan that's very large for our size. Not that we always use all the intelligence we have – especially when we do things we know we shouldn't, like bending over to lift heavy objects or slouching for hours in front of the TV.

Our bones are surrounded by myriad soft tissues, some of which link the bones to one another, others that keep them from painfully rubbing together (as in arthritis), and still others that actuate your bones' movements. Collectively, these are called connective tissue.

The tissue that cushions the ends of bones, for example in the hip joint between your pelvis and thigh bone (or femur), or in the knee between the femur and the tibia and fibula bones below, is called cartilage. It provides elasticity and direction for movement, allowing us to twist and pivot when driving a golf ball or to turn around to look at the baby in the back seat.

Cartilage also provides structure for many parts of the body, such as the nose, which is more cartilage than bone; it also keeps our rib cage in line, among many other functions. And, unfortunately, it has a way of wearing out from years of use or becoming damaged through some type of injury, sometimes requiring that a whole hip, knee or elbow be replaced to relieve pain and restore movement.

Ligaments work in conjunction with cartilage, tying the bones together and helping guide their motion so we can walk, sink a foul shot, volley on the tennis court or type words on a keyboard. We don't think about ligaments much until we strain them beyond their limits, even painfully tearing them in ways that can require surgery and physical therapy. Skiing and playing soccer are two sports where a common injury is a tear of the ACL, or anterior cruciate ligament, which often leads to the operating room, crutches and a long period of recovery.

Tendons tie bones to muscles, and are the drive train for all our movement in a way that today's engineers and roboticists are forever trying to imitate and perfect.

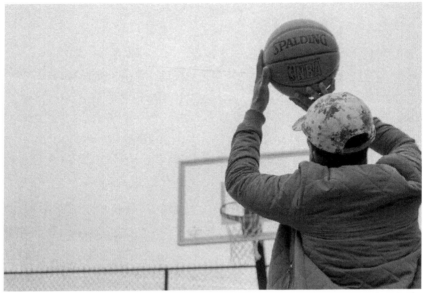

Photo by Tamarcus Brown on Unsplash

It's an ingenious system:

Muscles in your forearm, linked by tendons to the bones in your hand, flex, extend and pivot your wrist up and down.

Muscles in your upper arm, linked to the bones in your forearm, let you raise and drop your lower arm.

And tendons connecting the forearm muscles to the bone in your upper arm near the elbow let you twist your forearm up, down and sideways so you can throw a ball overhanded or underhanded, put spin on your tennis serve or swing a bat to hit a home run.

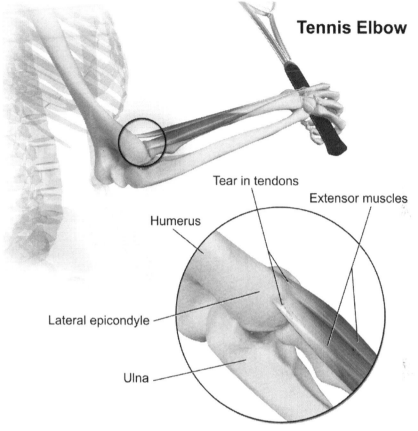

Tennis Elbow

Tear in tendons

Extensor muscles

Humerus

Lateral epicondyle

Ulna

Bruce Blaus
Blausen.com staff (2014).
"Medical gallery of Blausen Medical 2014".
WikiJournal of Medicine 1 (2).
DOI:10.15347/wjm/2014.010. ISSN 2002-4436

But of course, like cartilage and ligaments, tendons are subject to injury from overstretching and over-stressing. "Tennis elbow," for example, is a chronic condition often caused by repetitive overexertion of the arm muscles, leading to injuries of the extensor tendon. These injuries often fail to heal properly because of continued strain on the extensor muscles. Scar tissue and adhesions form and the pain and accompanying weakness can last for months or even years.

Sudden injuries, such as a tear in a crucial structure like the Achilles Tendon, which ties your calf muscles to your foot providing power and stability for standing, walking and running, are common in the connective tissue as well. Often sports-related but sometimes caused by something simple like misjudging a step on the staircase, a tear in the Achilles Tendon is a painful and debilitating injury that again often requires an orthopedic surgeon to rectify.

FASCIA

Another type of connective tissue exists virtually everywhere in the body, holding parts of us together, providing pathways for blood and lymphatic vessels and nerves, and lubricating the movements of our muscles and other tissues. This is fascia, and for compelling reasons it is the nexus of a Naprapathic treatment.

Fascia is a tough connective tissue that spreads

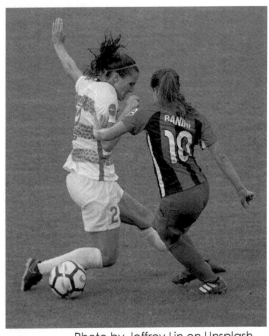

Photo by Jeffrey Lin on Unsplash

14

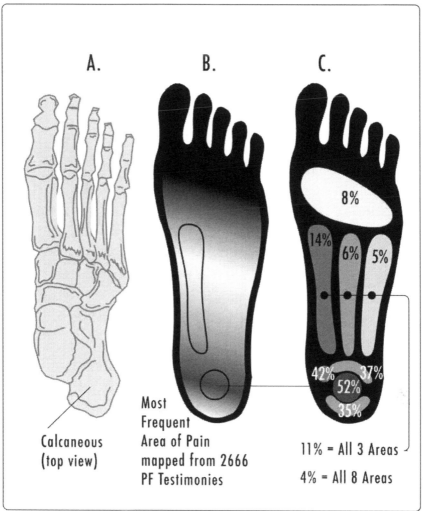

A.

Calcaneous
(top view)

B.

Most
Frequent
Area of Pain
mapped from 2666
PF Testimonies

C.

8%

14%

6% 5%

42% 37%

52%

35%

11% = All 3 Areas

4% = All 8 Areas

One segment of human fascia unfortunately familiar to many people is the Plantar Fascia -- rugged tissue under the skin at the bottom of the foot that can be come inflamed and painful. This illustration shows where many sufferers feel Plantar Fasciitis pain.

Wiliikepedia illustration by Kosigrim,
Llcensed under Creative Commons

throughout the body in a three-dimensional web from your head to your feet, without interruption. In form and function, it is sometimes compared to an intricate spider web or closely knit sweater. As you study the fascia, you can begin to see that each part of the body is connected to every other by this ubiquitous tissue.

Despite its ruggedness – in parts of your body such as the hip and thigh having the tensile strength of steel – it appears as thin, membranous and nearly transparent. In function, it bends when it needs to, holds tight when it needs to, covers and protects physical structures in the body, and lets one muscle slide along another to give us the desired motion of our limbs and trunk. When examined in a normal, healthy state, the fascia is wavy and relaxed in configuration, complementing the structures to which it is attached. It has the ability to stretch and move without restriction.

Fascia, though, is overlooked in most studies of injury and disease – except when it stops working like it's supposed to. Trauma or inflammation from an injury such as whiplash, or a fall, surgery, repetitive stress and more, can affect fascia, creating a binding down that results in excessive pressure on nerves, muscles, blood vessels, osseous structures (bones) and/or organs.

The standard diagnostic tests such as x-rays, myelograms, electromyography, CAT scans and MRIs do not show fascial restrictions, though broken bones and torn ligaments and tendons tend to be easily visualized and diagnosed. Thus, in the absence of injury to another body structure, it is thought that an extremely high percentage of people suffering with pain, headaches and/or lack of motion may be having problems from fascia that has become bound and inflexible.

But most go undiagnosed. Oftentimes the role of the fascia in a patient's symptoms is misunderstood or ignored by traditional medicine. Yet, it is here that Naprapathic intervention can play a vital role in treatment and recovery from an often debilitating condition.

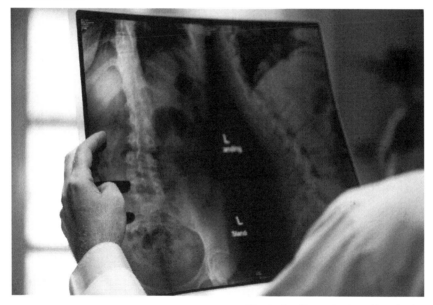

Photo by Rawpixel on Unsplash

Naprapathy allows the practitioner to look at each patient as a unique individual. Therapy sessions are hands-on treatments during which doctors use a multitude of techniques and movement therapy to drive away pain and return the body to normal function.

The goal of Naprapathy is to restore the individual's myofascial freedom so they may return to a pain-free, active lifestyle.

CHAPTER TWO

YOUR FIRST VISIT TO A NAPRAPATHIC PHYSICIAN

When you first visit a Naprapathic physician, your practitioner will be evaluating many things, including the symptoms you describe, signs such as a limp or limited motion, the relative positions of your pelvis and shoulders (is one side lower than the other), and your stance – are you bending to one side or the other when you stand or sit; is your head tilted off the centerline?

He or she will note how you walk into the treatment room, the strength of your grip while shaking hands, your posture, even your smile – or lack thereof if you are in pain. You will also answer some questions to give your doctor a comprehensive history of the problem that brought you to the Naprapathic physician, as well as other relevant medical details.

It is all part of a whole body diagnosis process that is at the heart of a Naprapathic treatment. Your practitioner of course wants to know the answer to that most basic of all medical questions, "Where does it hurt?" But beyond that painful expression of illness or injury lies the cause, and that is what requires treatment.

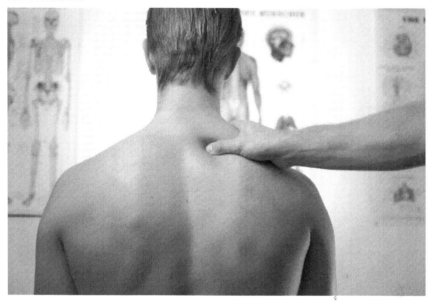

Photo by Jesper Aggergaard on Unsplash

Pain is not always what it seems. It may spread out from the injury, masking the true source. It can also occur elsewhere in the body, seemingly unrelated to what actually is causing you to hurt. A heart attack, for example, can cause pain in your neck, back or shoulders. If it manifests in conjunction with chest pain, the more distant discomfort is called radiating pain. If there is pain elsewhere but not in the chest, it is known as referred pain.

This somewhat illogical transfer of the pain from one part of your body to another is very commonly seen in musculoskeletal conditions as well. We know of one man, a marathoner who went to an orthopedic

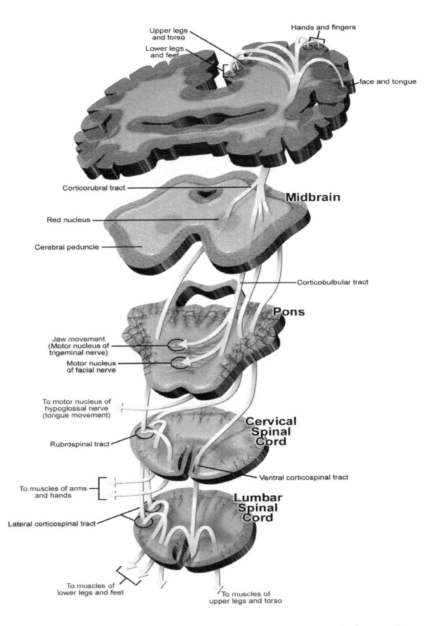

Motor nerve pathways carry commands from the brain, down the spinal cord and throughout the body.

Bruce Blaus, Blausen.com staff (2014). "Medical gallery of Blausen Medical 2014"WikiJournal of Medicine 1 (2). DOI:10.15347/wjm/2014.010. ISSN 2002-4436

physician complaining of knee pain. The orthopedist told him, "I'll bet it's your hip." And the examination showed that's exactly what it was.

Thus, your Naprapathic physician will ask you about your main complaint, but also about secondary complaints – those things you may not have focused on because other parts of you were hurting too much. It's a first step on the way to diagnosis and successful treatment.

Your doctor will ask about your occupation – whether you sit or stand most of the day, work at a computer or a construction site, lift and carry heavy objects or talk on the phone with your head bent for hours toward one or the other shoulder.

Is the pain deep? Burning (which indicates a nerve is part of the cause)? Stabbing? Dull or aching? Sharp (which points to a muscular origin)? How often does it occur? Is it constant, or only when you do certain things like bend over or type on a keyboard? How intense is the pain on a scale of 1 to 10, with 10 being the worst pain you can imagine?

What makes it better? Or worse? It could be the position of your body, perhaps slumping or sitting up straight. Maybe hot or cold relieves the pain. Maybe putting on the extra weight of safety gear brings the pain to the surface. Your Naprapathic physician will evaluate it all.

There's also the question of whether it was a sudden onset of the pain – did you fall, get rear-ended at a traffic light, feel it first when you lifted a heavy box or after catching an edge of your ski? Or did it manifest itself gradually and get worse over time?

Maybe you just don't know.

What does this pain prevent you from doing? This is one of the key questions, because it's often the most important factor in bringing a patient in for treatment.

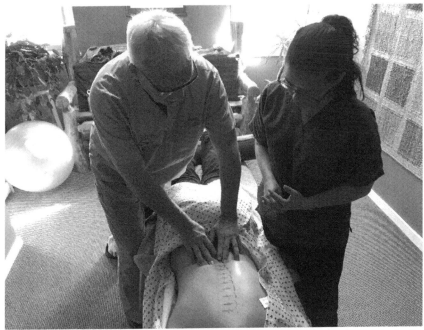

Dr. Kirsten LaVista/SUNM photo

Many people will tolerate pain to a certain point as long as it doesn't interfere with their preferred – or necessary – activities. But there is that moment when it gets in the way, when aspirin or ibuprofen no longer keeps it under control, when a sufferer says, "I've got to get help."

"Have you sought previous treatment?" is another important question, as is whether that treatment helped at all. Many people see a series of professionals hoping to find relief for their pain or disability – with greater or lesser success.

It's vital for your Naprapathic physician to know the

types of treatment you have had or believed you needed, and what was the result. You may have been to a chiropractor, your family doctor, a physical or massage therapist, a nutritionist or any of a dozen other medical and complementary alternative practices. Maybe something helped, but not enough. Maybe nothing worked. Maybe you feel that your true complaint wasn't addressed, even though some symptoms were treated.

Of course, it's essential for the Naprapathic physician to know about any courses of medication you've been on for this condition – as well as other prescription pharmaceuticals and non-prescription aids such as nutritional supplements or Non-Steroidal Anti-Inflammatory Drugs (NSAIDs) you may have taken or are currently taking. It's very common for people with musculoskeletal complaints to be prescribed steroids such as Prednizone, muscle relaxants and/or pain-killers ranging from Tylenol to Oxycontin. It will be important in your treatment to ascertain whether you actually need these drugs, or if Naprapathic Manual Medicine can make you better without them.

You also may be asked about supplements, vitamins and over-the-counter medications that you may be taking. There are countless products such as glucosamine advertising themselves as the cure for your joint pain. Your Naprapathic physician will help you determine if you need these supplements, if perhaps others would be beneficial, or if you should stay away from certain touted "remedies" completely because they'll do you more harm than good.

Your diet and your liquid intake will also be of interest to the doctor. We all know that some foods are good for you and some not so good, but sometimes we're not that great at eating the right foods. Your Naprapathic physician may spot something in your diet that is contributing to your condition, or may recommend certain foods and nutrients because they're likely to help.

Liquids are not all created equal. Though virtually everything we drink is made mostly of water – that indispensible ingredient of life – the other chemicals, substances and compounds in a particular liquid may not be so desirable. We'll discuss this further in a following chapter. Meanwhile, drink purified water, it's good for you.

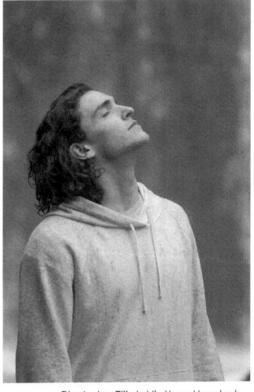

Allergies are another issue. It's not as simple as sneezing when there's pollen in the air. In fact, allergic reactions to dust or

Photo by Elijah Hiett on Unsplash

certain foods or other substances we commonly encounter are actually an overreaction of the immune system to those generally harmless substances. And, of course, the resulting inflammation can be deadly, in some cases constricting the throat or swelling the tongue so you can't breathe. Your Naprapathic physician might ask about allergies because they could, without your realizing it, be causing distress that at casual glance would seem unrelated.

Family history is another factor that may play a role and prompt a question. If your grandmother had sciatica and you have sciatic pain and limited motion, your Naprapathic physician will know there is a need to focus on the nerves affecting your lower back and leg on the troubled side. Where the sciatic nerve

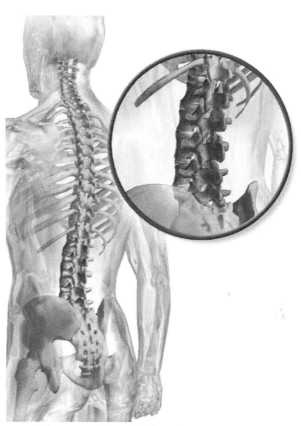

The Lumbar Spine is composed of the vertebrae in the lower back.

Blausen.com staff (2014). "Medical gallery of Blausen Medical 2014". WikiJournal of Medicine 1 (2). DOI:10.15347/wjm/2014.010. ISSN 2002-4436.

emerges from the spinal column, at the fourth and fifth lumbar vertebrae, is a common site for adhesions and constrictions that lead to pain and movement problems in your leg and foot. And it runs in families.

Then there are accidents (with resulting trauma) and surgeries, which can cause the type of painful, limiting conditions for which many people seek out manual medicine. It's essential that the doctor know about any of these as they can pinpoint where and how to treat your complaint.

Do you exercise, and how much/often? Exercise can both help and hurt, and your Naprapathic physician will look at this as both a potential component of your

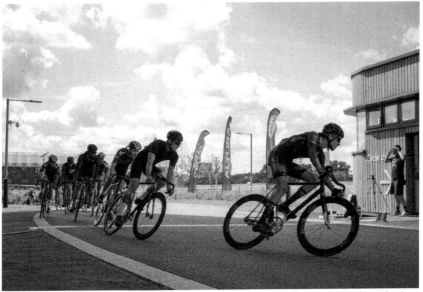

Photo by Yomex Owo on Unsplash

distress and a possible part of your treatment. You may take home suggestions for keeping your connective tissues loose and limber such as stretching over an exercise ball.

Do you sleep well? Sleep through the night? What position(s) do you sleep in? How many pillows and what kind of support do they give your head and neck? Do you sit up to read, watch TV or work on your iPad in bed? All can have an influence on your physical well-being.

It may seem like a lot of questions if your complaint is shoulder pain or a crick in your lower back, but Naprapathy treats the whole person, and as we've seen, everything inside you is connected in some way to everything else. If you're nervous that you'll forget things when talking to the doctor, write it down, make a list of your questions and concerns. Your diagnosis and resulting treatment will be that much better for it.

CHAPTER THREE

WHAT WE'RE MADE OF

Fascia, as we've seen, is everywhere in the body, surrounding every muscle and every bone, connecting organs to surrounding structure, letting things slip and slide where they need to and holding them together to give the body shape and function.

And, we've noted, fascia also surrounds our neurovascular bundles. These vital anatomical structures thread blood and lymphatic vessels throughout the body to bring messages from the brain directing various organs and muscles to do their stuff, and they also bring nourishment from the heart, lungs and digestive system so our many billions of cells can fuel the fires for the whole human organism.

Fascia has not been viewed in traditional medical thinking as a bodily system dedicated to unique functions as are our livers, lungs or kidneys, but Naprapathy has long recognized that it in fact works hand-in-hand with the lymphatic and other systems to perform a number of dedicated and vital tasks.

Finally, however, modern medical science has begun to come around with the discovery of a "new" organ, dubbed the "Interstitium," that in fact is the body-wide fascial system that Dr. Oakley Smith focused his attentions on more than a century ago, and that Naprapathic Physicians have been treating ever since.

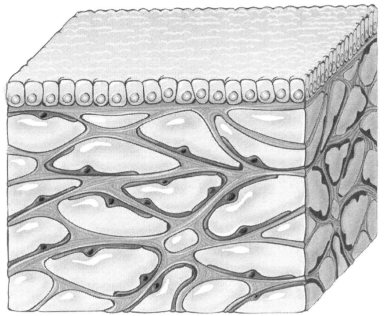

Interstitium illustration by Jill Gregory
Mount Sinai Health System
Licensed under Creative Commons.

What is bringing the medical establishment around is the visualization for the first time, using a new diagnostic imaging technique, of fluid-filled channels running through the connective tissue. These channels were previously thought to be solid, but now are recognized as conduits. As Tom Myers explains in his anatomytrains.com blog, the Interstitium "is a body-wide communicating system for the push and pull of mechanical information. A system of collagen and elastin fibres suspended in a mucousy gel that binds with interstitial (inter-cellular) fluid, this system is closely aligned with the lymphatic system and the white blood cells of the immune system."[1]

It is part of the fascial system that Naprapaths and others who treat soft tissue have long addressed in their practices, and provides the additional benefits of cushioning organs against outside forces and usually springs back where it belongs when the force is removed.

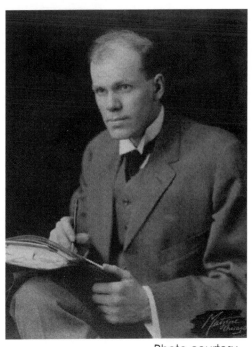

Photo courtesy
of Jeff B. Smith

Dr. Oakley Smith

However, as Dr. Smith found, fascia and surrounding tissue that suffer injuries can scar and get bound up, preventing free flow of the fluids that power its work, as well as limiting movement and causing pain. Treating this involves applying pressure to free up the strictures, along with stretching and other manipulation of the connective tissue (sometimes called "myofascial release") to restore

---

[1] https://www.anatomytrains.com/blog/2018/03/29/interstitium-statement-tom-myers/

flow and function, as well as relieve discomfort.

Why is this necessary? Let's get back to what we're made of and how our bodies work.

Our lymph vessels are routed through the fascia, using the action of the fascial tissue as our muscles expand and contract to assist their work in draining fluid from organs and muscles and returning it to the circulatory system.

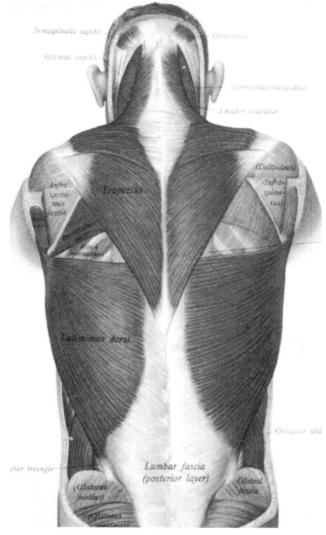

A 1914 illustration of the back shows the large lumbar fascia.

Atlas and Text-Book of Human Anatomy. Johannes Sobotta, J. Playfair McMurrich; Publisher: Saunders Philadelphia.

Much of our metabolic waste is transmitted through the lymph vessels to the various organs that process and get rid of the things that we don't need. We'll discuss this more in another chapter. For now, remember that our bodies are 78 percent water – and have a sip of some healthy, purified H2O.

The lymph system is also a primary transitway working on behalf of our immune system – something

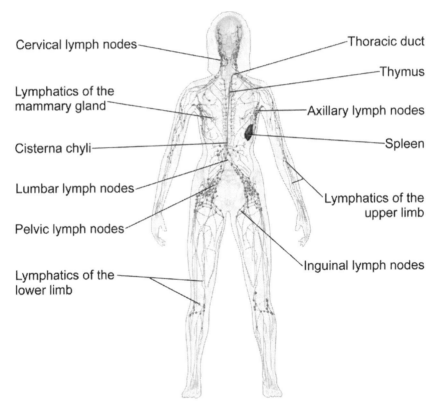

Cervical lymph nodes

Thoracic duct

Thymus

Lymphatics of the mammary gland

Axillary lymph nodes

Cisterna chyli

Spleen

Lumbar lymph nodes

Lymphatics of the upper limb

Pelvic lymph nodes

Inguinal lymph nodes

Lymphatics of the lower limb

Blausen.com staff (2014). "Medical gallery of Blausen Medical 2014". WikiJournal of Medicine 1 (2). DOI:10.15347/wjm/2014.010. ISSN 2002-4436

we stop to consider only when our lymph nodes get swollen because of an infectious disease such as the mumps. Our lymph nodes are in reality organic arsenals teeming with lymphocytes, the immune cells that often form the front lines against internal and external foes, such as bacteria and viruses.

Lymphocytes are also deployed by the body to divert the multiplicity of toxins around us from causing harm,

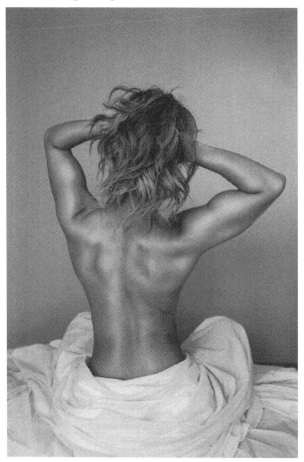

and are active in seeking out and doing battle with cancerous cells as well. Many researchers believe that cancers would be forming in our bodies all the time if it weren't for the immune system hunting down cells that are dangerously mutating and eliminating them before they divide wildly into a tumor.

Shayla Edenfield Photography

To do its job, the lymphatic system needs to be free-flowing, just the way that the nervous system must be without blockages and constrictions if it's to properly do the brain's bidding. The binding and adhesions that make our backs hurt or our repetitively stressed hands get stiff and numb also affect the operation of the lymph vessels, and thus affect the body's ability to get rid of waste and fight disease. Manual medicine as practiced by Naprapathic Physicians is aimed at freeing up these vital pathways in a treatment that may be first aimed at relieving pain and restoring function, but also is designed to improve whole body health. A healthy lymphatic system is absolutely essential to our well-being.

Note that Naprapathy aims to enhance our health, not merely treat the symptom that bring people to the doctor. Thus derives the focus on the back and spine, where these bundles of nerves, lymphatic and blood vessels originate. Freeing them up at the source is what relieves conditions that appear elsewhere, such as sciatica, which manifests as pain and paralysis in the legs but is caused by constriction and misalignment in the spine or piriformis muscle.

And the benefits, according to recent research, show up in interesting and positive ways. It is now understood that focusing on exercise that works our nerve pathways builds better strength and conditioning than just doing the reps at the gym. The new advice in strength-building, for example, is to push harder and work our muscles to the limit rather than to do more reps with less weight or resistance. Fewer but heavier is the formula that stimulates the nerves to tell the brain that we're trying to build strength in a particular part of the body.

This kind of training is changing the way we work out – and improving the results we get. In fact, the growing science of sports medicine is contributing greatly to our knowledge of the body's systems and how they work. If you look at a professional sports team, the roster includes medical doctors such as orthopedists,

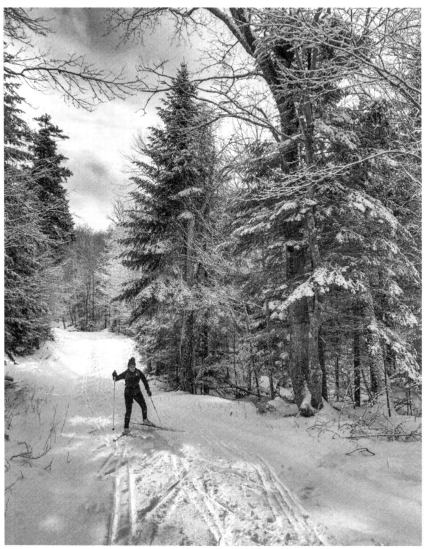

Photo by Philip Belena on Unsplash

physiologists and physiatrists (more about these specialties later), nutritionists, physical trainers, massage therapists and others who practice forms of manual manipulation and treatment, to keep the athletes in good health and top physical shape.

Several well-known professional teams in the U.S. and Scandinavia have brought Naprapathic Physicians on board to benefit from their unique knowledge and methods of treating soft tissue. The *Routledge Handbook of Sports Event Management* (Routledge, 2015), in an analysis of the FIS Nordic World Ski Championships in 2011 written by Elsa Kristiansen, Glyn C. Roberts and Pierre-Nicolas Lemyre of the Norwegian School of Sport Sciences, notes that an

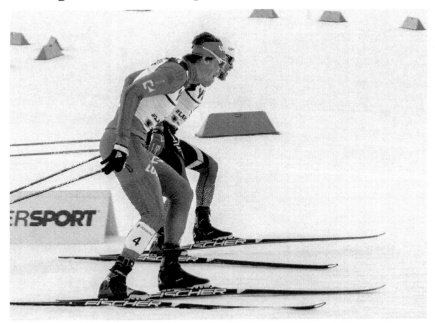

Photo by Martine Jacobsen on Unsplash

athlete's "entourage," along with several skiing coaches, two ski waxers and an endurance expert, also included a "mental coach" and a Naprapath.

There is no question that athletes and team leaders

understand the whole body nature of health – that it is not merely flexing and strengthening muscles that determines performance, but rather the smooth synchronization of all the systems in the body. These systems communicate via the bundles buried in our fascia, and when those are constricted the ability to perform at our peak is diminished.

Within these bundles that originate at the spine, nerves that are free and unrestricted transmit messages to the muscles and organs more efficiently, while likewise unhindered lymph vessels quickly carry away the metabolic waste generated by our activities, and unconstrained blood vessels bring the nutrition that it takes to build stronger muscle cells.

As you see, the whole body approach of Naprapathy fits right in with these cutting-edge methods of making ourselves healthier and happier, and able to be our best.

CHAPTER FOUR

THERE'S NO SHORTAGE
OF STRESS

Think of your body as a sailboat. Your spine is the mast, your muscles are the sails, and your connective tissues are the lines that hold the mast

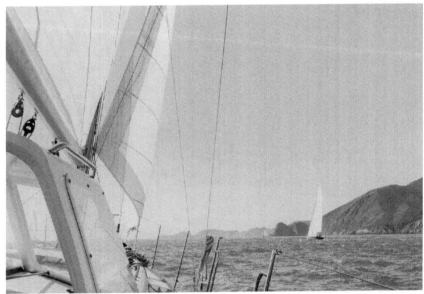

Photo by Milkovi on Unsplash

and the sails together.

In a boat on the water, if there's no wind the sails hang limp, held at the ready by the combined structure of the mast and lines, but exerting no force on them. Your boat stands upright and makes no way.

Add a breeze and the sail begins to fill, putting tension on the lines and readying your craft for action. The wind picks up and your boat starts to move, the force exerted on the sails transmitted through the lines and the mast, pushing you forward. At the same time, it heels, or leans away from the wind, pulled off the vertical by the physics of force meeting the structure. Watch the way a sprinter leans forward in a 100-yard dash to see a body adapting to this type of force.

If the wind grows strong, your boat leans sharply abeam as its forward speed grows. Too strong and instead of forward progress, the wind energy pushes the boat to the side so hard it threatens to capsize or break the mast – unless the sailors compensate by letting up on the lines, changing the center of gravity by moving to the high side of the deck or even stretching their bodies over the waves, or steering the boat so the gale puts less stress on the structure.

In your body, the muscles provide the force, which is transmitted to your bony structure by the connective tissues. When everything works right, you are smoothly sailing forward, the force and the structure in equilibrium and getting done what you have to do. Too much force and you can do the equivalent of capsizing or damaging the mast, even pulling spinal vertebrae out of place or tearing soft tissue.

You can also foul the lines – on a boat by mishandling and getting a knot or kink in the lines or damaging a block; in your body by chronic stress in your muscles pulling the connective tissue out of place or pinching the bundles of nerves, blood and lymph vessels and inhibiting their free function.

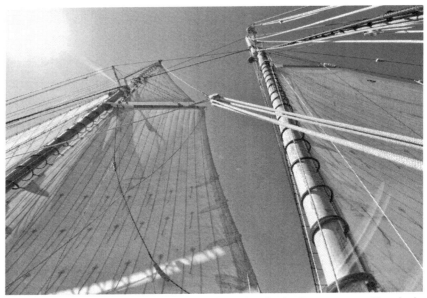

Photo by Craig Cameron on Unsplash

There is no shortage of stress in our modern lives, and some of it is very good stress. Physical stress allows us to work, stay alert, exercise, pick up a cup of coffee – or our kids. Stressing our muscles builds strength and stressing our connective tissue builds agility – much of the time. Of course, overstressing our muscles and connective tissue – say that day you decide to get healthy and take the five flights of stairs to your office for the first time, or when the weekend warrior in you spends a day hammering and sawing when you hardly ever hammer and saw – causes pain, though it usually gets better with a few days' rest.

We all have psychological stress at times, some of us handling it better than others, and again it usually goes away when the trigger eases up – a deadline at work, relationship problems, grief for a lost parent or friend, or exiting a stressful environment like military combat. But sometimes these psychological stresses remain when the trigger is gone and cause a myriad of physical difficulties.

With psychological stress, your brain and body pump out neurotransmitters such as norepinephrine that keep us alert and at the ready for action. These in turn trigger hormones like cortisol, which primes our muscles and gets us ready to fight or flee (known as the "Fight or Flight Response"). At these times our personal boat is heeling a bit; the stress pulling on our mast even though we're not moving forward.

This stress gives us head and muscle aches, strains our backs, numbs our feet and fingers and in general makes us miserable. Some of us suffer for years without relief despite our seeking all kinds of solutions, from pills to traction devices, and from aroma-heavy liniments to tricky surgeries. Psychological stress that manifests physically forces people to leave their jobs, halt their favorite activities and abdicate their lives. It ruins relationships. Causes disabling pain and discomfort. Drives us to drink or become addicted to harmful drugs.

Pain is not merely physical, but research reveals it also has a large psychological component. Being in pain physically provokes an emotional response as well — fear in many cases; depression when the pain is chronic; despair if nothing can make it go away.

The medical community is also recognizing that emotion can worsen pain, or make things that would not otherwise be uncomfortable become painful. But let's be clear, it's not "all in your mind" – it's how your mind is reacting, and again that goes back to the emotions you experience. It's a vicious circle that your Naprapathic Physician will team with you to break.

We discussed in detail the physical signs and symptoms the doctor will note during your first visit. Your psychological reaction to your physical issue is just as important, and is a vital consideration in your treatment. Indeed, the general question of "how do you feel" encompasses both your physical and psychological status, and you should be comfortable sharing with your Naprapathic Physician how the pain is affecting you emotionally as well as physically.

Musculoskeletal pain is not dangerous to life in and of itself, but the way we deal with it can be. The next chapter is devoted to opioids not because they are an answer for your pain, but because they can do much more harm than good. Among the thousands of deaths in the U.S. each year due to opioids are many people who began taking them as a heavily promoted and consequence-free solution to their problem. The result has been a sad and destructive epidemic of addiction and death.

The World Health Organization has called stress the "health epidemic of the 21st century." We agree. It needs to be addressed on an individual and societal basis, but it's not going to go away. People need access to help for their stress, and manual medicine is one modality that has been shown to work.

A pertinent example is Post-Traumatic Stress Disorder (PTSD) and its treatment. In 2012, urged on

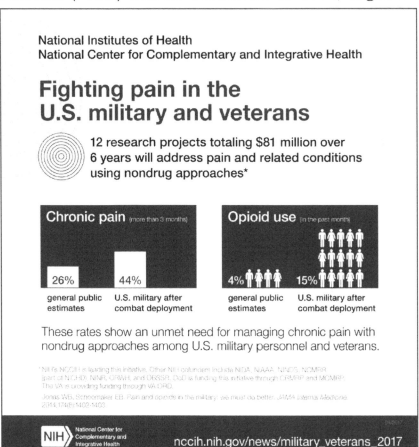

through a memorial passed by the Legislature of the State of New Mexico, the Southwest University of Naprapathic Medicine, conducted a preliminary survey of U.S. veterans who suffered from PTSD. Four women and five men – seven of whom were classed with a discernable level of disability due to chronic pain from their condition – received 10 weeks of Naprapathic treatment under the program. All nine showed some degree of pain relief, ranging from 10 to 90 percent.[2]

The survey also showed a significant decrease in "catastrophizing," or "the perception of devastation that can accompany physical pain associated with PTSD." Though small, the survey in addition showed a potential improvement in the quality of the patients' sleep. And on a scale of 1 to 10, the patients gave an average satisfaction score of 8.4 with the results of their Naprapathic treatment.

In the simplest of terms, these brave veterans who suffered ill effects from their service felt better after their visits to a Naprapathic physician – without drugs and without further disruption to their lives.

---

[2] SUNM Preliminary Survey on Veterans jointly affected by Musculoskeletal Pain and PTSD: BENEFITS OF NAPRAPATHIC MEDICINE ON VETERANS' HEALTH, Prepared by Dominique Alò, (Scientific Consultant for SUNM, Southwest University of Naprapathic Medicine)

CHAPTER FIVE

THE OPIOID CRISIS

A merica for the past two decades has been caught in a spiral of prescription drug addiction. As the successes of manual medicine demonstrate well, it did not have to be this way.

Opioid medications – those derived from the poppy plant – were long seen as a miracle for controlling pain. Those recovering from surgery, or who had suffered broken limbs, just undergone a root canal or were in the throes of acute pain caused by heart attacks and other medical emergencies were grateful to have fast, effective treatments for their agonizing symptoms. Their doctors, too, were for the most part happy that they could relieve their patients' suffering, but saw that these powerful drugs could be dangerous when used improperly.

Still, the tendency to prescribe them grew, spurred on by hard-sell marketing to medical doctors – who

should have known better – across the country.
Patients would, without even asking, many times be
handed a prescription for Vicodin or Percocet on the
way out the door after a doctor or dentist visit for a
relatively minor complaint. The intention was that the

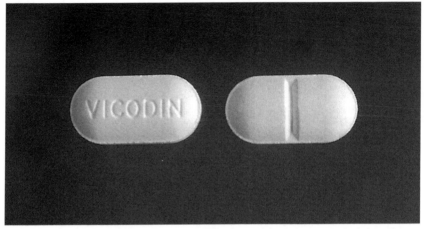

U.S. Drug Enforcement Administration

Vicodin tablets

medication would be taken for a few days or a week until
the acute back pain or tooth pain or whatever pain went
away, at which point the patient would feel well enough
to get by without any pills, or at most take over-the-
counter pain killers. There were addiction and overdose
problems, but when used as prescribed the drugs were
perceived as overwhelmingly safe and effective.

These fast-acting opioid medications did not fill
some patients' needs, however, and practitioners and
drug companies sought ways to manage chronic pain
such as that from musculoskeletal conditions – spinal
disc problems, sciatica, and other long-term issues that
plague the modern world. Their answer was the
development of timed-release opioid delivery systems

that would deliver small but effective doses to prevent pain for longer periods. Among the supposed benefits were that patients could still work, drive and function normally because the dosage would not hinder their cognitive or motor functions. One study that took place in Oregon, published in the Journal of the American Board of Family Medicine, looked at more than 26,000 patients with back pain. Sixty-one percent of them received a prescription for opioids during their treatment, and 19 percent took opioids on a long-term basis.

Indeed, it had been loudly pronounced by those hawking the drugs that people could use them as maintenance medications – like insulin or blood pressure pills – over the long term and suffer no ill effects.

For a number of reasons it did not work out that way. The Oregon study noted that, "The prevalence of psychologic distress, unhealthy lifestyles, and health care utilization increased incrementally with duration of use."[3]

Longer-term use often proved addicting. Many patients found the dosage inadequate and sought more of the drug. Plus, the timed-release delivery system was easily defeated by crushing a pill and getting a quick and powerful high from inhaling or injecting the now accessible opiate compound. Reports began to surface of rampant abuse of these supposedly safe medications, of rising crime including armed robberies of drug stores – and several times, sadly, the murders of pharmacists,

---

[3] http://www.jabfm.org/content/24/6/717.long

customers and clerks so a violent addict could obtain his opioid fix. In one horrific drug robbery on Long Island, New York, the perpetrator killed four people in a local drug store, including a 17-year-old clerk who was still in high school, two customers, one of them an elderly man, as well as the pharmacist.

JUST CALL THEM PUSHERS

Yet, the pharmaceutical companies spent untold millions to market these heavily profitable drugs, even though it later emerged that they knew of the problems being caused by pills like Oxycontin, which brought its manufacturer billions of dollars in income every year. The incomprehensible reaction of Purdue Pharma when the pressure to change its ways was initially applied was to launch a "campaign against pain," including high-pressure marketing to physicians, a sophisticated website urging patients to request the drug, and publicly blaming those who had used their drug as prescribed yet fallen victim to its addictive nature. Many of these patients – middle-class working people, family people, churchgoers – had taken an opioid after surgery or for another indicated use, complied with the instructions from their doctors, but still became desperate addicts who would do anything to secure more of the drug.

The drug companies became nothing more than "pushers," serving up dangerous narcotics to people in distress and profiting mightily in the process. They brought about overdose deaths and deaths from violent crime, splintered families, ruined the lives of young and old alike, and only when forced by the law and changing public opinion began to back off from their unconscionable and tragic trafficking of lethal danger in the form of a "miraculous" white pill. Purdue Pharma announced early in 2018, after more than a decade of public pressure, that its sales force would stop visiting doctors to promote Oxycontin.[4]

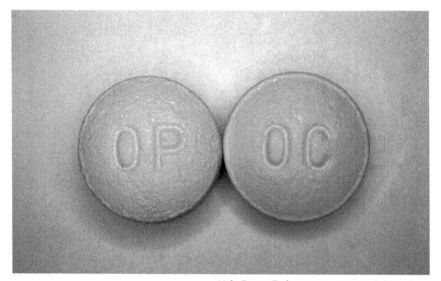

U.S. Drug Enforcement Administration

Oxycontin pills

Opiates are neither the best nor the only treatments for pain, a fact that gradually dawned on the country over the past 15 years and has begun to alter the pain management landscape. Manual medicine such as Naprapathy has been demonstrated to be effective in treating pain by manipulating ligaments, tendons and fascia to facilitate spinal alignment. Evidence is mounting that such successful pain treatment greatly

[4] https://www.bloomberg.com/news/articles/2018-02-10/pain-pill-giant-purdue-to-stop-promotion-of-opioids-to-doctors?mod=article_inline

reduces stress – even the effects of PTSD, which troubles so many of our brave veterans.

In fact, the survey by the Southwest University of Naprapathic Medicine with a group of veterans suffering PTSD showed that patients in the survey suffering chronic pain as a result of their condition felt some degree of relief ranging from 10 percent to 90 percent after a course of Naprapathic therapy. Psychologically, patients who had lost hope that they were ever going to feel better felt more positive at the end of the survey, and showed increasing satisfaction with the results of their treatment.

Contrast this with a recent study by the Minneapolis Veterans Health Care System that opioids were no better in treating lower back pain than over-the-counter NSAIDs like aspirin, ibuprofen or acetaminophen. In fact, 12 months after beginning treatment the patients prescribed opioids had more pain and no more improvement in function than patients who didn't get the addictive drugs.[5]

RETIRING THE OPIOID MODALITY

Today, many in the medical field have turned away from the liberal prescribing of opioid medicines and more toward therapies that are natural and safe. For musculoskeletal conditions, manual therapies have proven a highly effective alternative to drugs, with a greater likelihood of returning an individual to an active

[5]https://journals.lww.com/backletter/Citation/2017/07000/Landmark_Trial_Punctures_the_Myth_That_Opioids.1.aspx

and productive life while avoiding disability and deleterious side effects.

Sure, it seems easier and cheaper to give a patient a prescription than to prescribe a course of physical treatment. In the long run, however, the costs have become clearer – for the individual, the healthcare system, and society in general.

As a practitioner of Naprapathic medicine, I have seen time and again a patient go from functional disability and chronic, unmanageable pain to

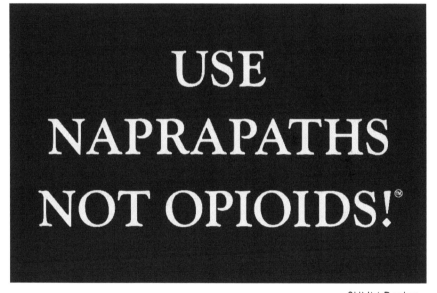

USE NAPRAPATHS NOT OPIOIDS!

SUNM Poster

productive work and renewed enjoyment of life. A course of manual treatment, of scientific, non-invasive, non-pharmaceutical therapy addressing of the cause of the condition, and not just the symptoms, has brought an individual back to her family, her job, her favorite activities and personal passions. Studies show that manipulative treatment for musculoskeletal pain helps the sufferer become more active, less disabled and more productive.

And consider this: If your Naprapathic treatment for pain, restricted movement and resulting stress, anxiety and depression does not include potentially addictive drugs, that treatment cannot make you an addict. That's a guarantee.

CHAPTER SIX

WATER, OXYGEN AND NUTRITION

W hen NASA tells the world that its astrometric instruments have found a distant planet that may sustain life, it really means one thing: That particular celestial body discovered so far from Earth might have liquid water on its surface, which is absolutely necessary for life as we know it to form.

If someone on another planet were taking the same type of scans looking at Earth, they'd see that the surface of our planet is about 71 percent water, a number that is similar to the amount of water contained in the human body. We begin life composed of as much as 78 percent water, and while we gradually have less as we age, we are always well more than half H_2O. Our bones are relatively dry at about 30 percent water, but some of our organs can measure well over 80 percent. More than 60 percent of the water in our bodies lies within our cells; the rest circulates outside the cells in our blood or lymphatic fluids, or in the various fluids that float around our organs, muscles and connective tissue.

DRINK

Water does many things for us, carrying nutrients to our muscles and life-sustaining systems and carting away our metabolic waste products. Within our cells, it facilitates the chemical interactions that make muscle cells contract, nerve cells fire their electric impulses, and skin cells retain their luster and flexibility.

As you probably remember from chemistry class, water is a solvent, meaning that other substances can be diluted and held in solution by water. You may see instructions for certain pills that say to take them with a full glass of water. Often, this is to dilute their contents so they are more easily absorbed by the body. Sometimes it is to cushion their impact on the digestive system, which may be upset by too strong a concentration of certain substances. If you've ever reached for a glass of water after biting into a green chili cheeseburger or a hot buffalo wing, you know the effect. Emergency medical personnel are taught to treat exposure to certain toxic substances, such as bleach or acid, first and foremost with plenty of water to quickly stop the harmful reactions.

For our discussion of Naprapathy, we will focus on several properties of water that affect our body's motion and our connective tissue. The first is a property that we all know from the shower, driving our car in the rain, or picking up a glass covered in condensation. It's "slippery when wet," like the road signs say. Water is, in certain circumstances, a lubricant, easing the friction between two surfaces in contact with each other. If

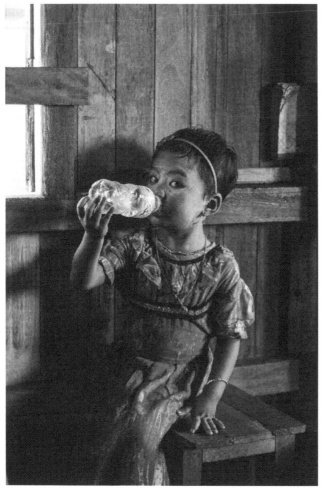

Photo by Chine Le Luc on Unsplash

you've ever been on a waterslide, you get the idea. Fiberglass and skin usually exhibit quite a bit of friction when one is drawn across the other, but add some water and suddenly you're zipping down the slide into the pool.

Dutch scientists discovered that water acts as a lubricant on a molecular level, speeding up the action of microscopic machines and potentially can be seen as "life's lubricant."[6] Water was able to stabilize – in effect smooth the surface of –these machines and ease their work, while other solvents they tried bonded with the molecules and slowed them down. It wasn't exactly like putting oil in your car or lubricating a squeaky door, but it did the job. Their research showed that water may do the same for enzymes and biological molecules – the building blocks of life.

As we noted above, water is present within and outside the billions of organic cells that make up the human body, and our insides are pretty slippery because of it. For one muscle to slide easily along another, and for the tendons that hold muscle to bone to do the same, they need lubrication, which water-based biologic fluids provide. Fascia, which is everywhere in the body, likewise need these lubricating fluids so they don't bind up and hamper our motion.

Dehydration, the common problem of people who are doing physical labor or working out, makes it more difficult for our bodies to do what we ask of them, and can lead to muscle aches and cramps – and even to severe systemic dysfunction and death. According to the Mayo Clinic, the loss of even 1 percent of our body's water can result in multiple ill effects, including feeling tired, weak and headachy, and cause our organs to go into a defensive mode that prevents us from keeping up that level of activity. Water is a key ingredient in

[6] https://www.chemistryworld.com/news/water-acts-as-a-lubricant-for-molecular-machines/6538.article

maintaining our body temperature, an essential life function that facilitates everything we do, from running a mile to mowing the lawn to thinking about the book we're reading.

Maybe you've heard the athletes' slogan, "Hydrate or Die!" It's a fact; we have to supply our bodies with water continually to keep ourselves going. Do it with good, purified water, and your body will do the rest.

Why purified water? Well, first, going back to the Dutch scientists, they found that other substances became bound with the tiny machines they were observing and hampered their work. The structures in our body that Naprapathy endeavors to treat and heal are very much like little machines. Second, water is the solvent that carries nutrition to our cells and within our cells, and nutrition is best when it is natural and not adulterated by unneeded and unwanted impurities.

BREATHE

If you want to light a fire under yourself, breathe!

Just as water is indispensable to life and the human body, so too is the air that we breathe. We are walking, talking, chemical-processing plants that take raw materials from our environment and convert them into energy. Oxygen is the key to making it all happen. And it does so in a reaction very much akin to what happens when we touch a match to a piece of paper in the fireplace. David Kahana, a Brookhaven National Laboratory physicist, called it "a highly controlled process of burning our food."[7]

When we eat, the acids in our digestive system break down the various food molecules into many components such as sugars and starches. These are the raw materials for our body's cells to function. Within the cells, a chemical process using oxygen from our bloodstream extracts energy from these molecules to power the cell's function – whether it's thinking, giving motion to your legs or causing your heart to beat.

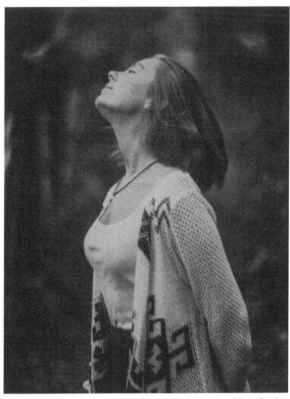

Photo by Valentina Alexandrovna on Unsplash

In the lungs, our blood is oxygenated through the dozen or so breaths we take every minute. When we exhale, the gaseous waste product of our cellular metabolism, carbon dioxide, is removed from our bodies. Likewise, excess water from our cells' energy-making activities is excreted via the kidneys.

It is an elegant system that depends on all the

---

[7] https://www.quora.com/What-purpose-does-oxygen-have-for-the-human-body-and-how-does-it-affect-the-body

necessary ingredients being present at the right time and in the right quantities. It's somewhat like a smoothly functioning auto factory where the parts are conveyed to the correct place on the assembly line while the workers supply the energy to put them together.

So where does breathing – something we do so automatically we rarely think about it – enter into the realm of Naprapathy? The answer lies in the whole health nature of the practice. Naprapathy, as we know, doesn't look only at the muscles and connective tissue, but sees the human body as an integrated system in which all parts must be working in harmony to keep us well.

Breathing manifests in many forms: slow and rhythmic when we're at rest or asleep; short and rushed if we're tense; deep if we're about to dive under water; huffing and puffing if we've just run a mile. Most of these scenarios are controlled by our autonomic nervous system, which is tasked, like a factory manager, with keeping all the processes going. However, we can also in many circumstances control our breathing. It's a basic exercise in yoga; singers and athletes are taught how to do it in order to improve their performance; people with anxiety causing a perceived shortness of breath are coached in ways to relax and breath normally.

Any of these methods of breath control – and perhaps all of them – may be appropriate for some who seek Naprapathic treatment. At the very least, we all should try to keep active, exercise enough to breathe heavily a few times a week, and keep our bodies functioning at their best.

EAT

We read lot about nutrition, especially when it comes to children and raising them to be strong, healthy adults. Our bodies need a large variety of

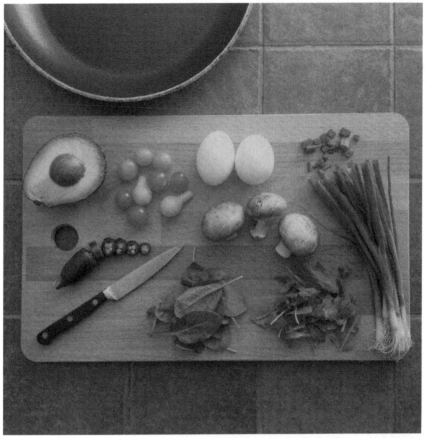

Photo by Katie Smith on Unsplash

nutrients – proteins, carbohydrates, vitamins and minerals – which we normally supply ourselves by eating vegetables, dairy products, meat and fish, grains in bread and pasta – and other foods that may not be so great, like excesses of sugars and fats.

Many people stick to certain diets that they believe are good for them, and for many conditions a diet that

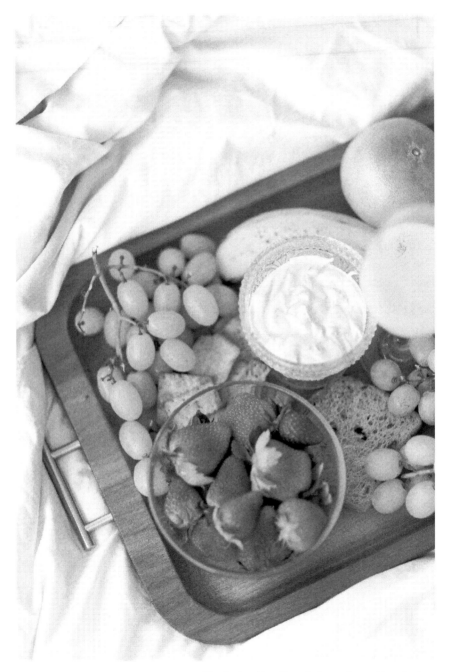

Photo by Heather Schwartz on Unsplash

emphasizes or leaves out some items is just what the

doctor ordered. If you have a heart condition, you don't want to eat bacon every day; if you have celiac disease, grains such as barley, wheat and rye will cause painful and debilitating digestive symptoms.

For the most part, however, we can eat a balanced diet and maintain our health. The question is what forms a balanced diet, and what do we need to ingest to keep at the top of our game. As you've probably heard, a balanced diet usually obviates the need for vitamins and supplements by giving us the raw materials that contain them before they are processed into pills and powders. Did you know that we make our own vitamin D? All it takes is getting the appropriate amount of sunlight and the exquisite chemical machine that is the human body manufactures what we require. (Note, though, that in northern climes it is hard to get the necessary amount of sun to spur the reaction, and wherever we live we don't want to overdo it.)

Most other vitamins and minerals are supplied to the body from outside, through eating well. What does that mean?

- Fresh, fresh, fresh.
- Farm to table.
- Doing the bulk of our shopping in the produce aisle (or farmers market if available) and avoiding the freezer case.
- Choosing seasonal fruits and vegetables and avoiding highly processed foods. (bagged, canned, boxed)
- Cooking dinner on the stove rather than in the microwave.

- If you're going to eat beef, pork or chicken, make sure it's organic, pasture-raised and grass-fed.

- Choosing meat and eggs without hormones and antibiotics.

- Choosing fish that is wild-caught rather than farm-raised.

- Enjoying our meals not only for their flavor but the fact that we made them from ingredients that we bought and prepared ourselves, rather than the factory kitchen thousands of miles away.

- We don't necessarily need that "daily vitamin," though certainly we should listen to our bodies and our doctors and make sure we're not causing ourselves any deficiencies of needed nutrients.

Does it mean we can't enjoy a hot dog at a picnic, or a slice of pepperoni pizza? Of course not, but we also realize that in our daily diet we shouldn't eat any highly processed foods – or the fast foods available on every corner in today's world.

For the bulk of human history, there were no such things as processed foods, no preservatives, no "ready to eat" from a can or frozen package. The human body is built from natural elements that are amazingly formed into bones and muscles and organs – and connective tissue – and work together in harmony to give us rich, fulfilling lives.

The lesson? Eat well. Eat fresh. Eat a balanced diet. Don't overdo it, and don't worry needlessly. Give your body the right ingredients, and it will reward you with good health and abundant energy.

CHAPTER SEVEN

THE SCIENCE OF NAPRAPATHY

D r. Oakley Smith was a true disciple of the scientific method. Based on his clinical practice, treating thousands of patients with musculoskeletal pain and decreased function, he formed a theory of the cause – that it was the connective tissue of the body, constricted and limited in motion by injury, repetitive stress or other factors, that caused his patients unbearable agony and drove them to seek treatment.

Dr. Smith diligently did his research to locate evidence that his theory was correct, and as we recall from the introduction, found it in the laboratory, viewing x-rays and pathology samples that showed the fascia – binding nerves, blood and lymph vessels, and muscles – were likely at the root of their problems.

Manually treating his patients to free up the fascia from the strictures and adhesions that were causing dysfunction, he was able to reduce people's pain and restore their motion, setting them free to work and to

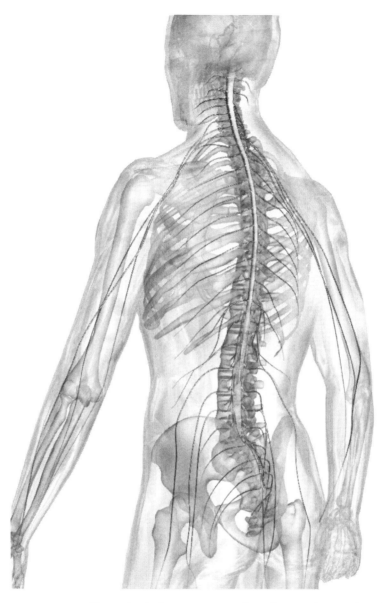

The dark lines emerging from the spine in this illustration represent the nerves that carry messages throughout the body.

Bruce Blaus, Blausen.com staff (2014). "Medical gallery of Blausen Medical 2014". WikiJournal of Medicine 1 (2). DOI:10.15347/wjm/2014.010. ISSN 2002-4436.

live their lives once again. And he was able to do it over and over again, fulfilling the scientific mandate that results be reproducible.

In the century-plus since Dr. Smith made his discoveries and launched the Naprapathic specialty, medicine has branched in many different directions, and great strides have been made in the treatment of countless diseases and conditions. Orthopedics in the latter half of the 20th century became one of the fastest growing medical disciplines as world populations aged and new techniques and technologies were explored to improve patients' lives. The first use of hip replacements dates to the 1960s[8], while knee replacements came along a decade later. Today, these are among the most-performed surgeries in the world.

However, these and other surgeries are not the ideal treatment for many patients. There are always the issues of risk, recovery and cost; some people are not surgical candidates because of age and other health conditions; there are other, less disruptive and less painful treatment modalities; and in many places patients have to wait months or longer, coping with pain and limitations on their activities, until they can have a procedure. Sometimes the condition will worsen during the wait. Additionally, some conditions simply do not lend themselves to surgical intervention – and often, the surgery won't help.

---

[8] Jackson, J. (2012). "Father of the modern hip replacement: Professor Sir John Charnley (1911-82)" *Journal of Medical Biography*. 19 (4): 151–156.

Twenty-first century medical researchers have thus trained their attention on alternative therapies to determine their efficacy in treating musculoskeletal conditions, when and how they should be used, and if they make patients' lives better.

Doctors in Sweden, where Naprapathy is a widely practiced manual medicine specialty, in 2010 published in the journal *Clinical Pain* a clinical trial report that had taken patients who were on waiting lists to see

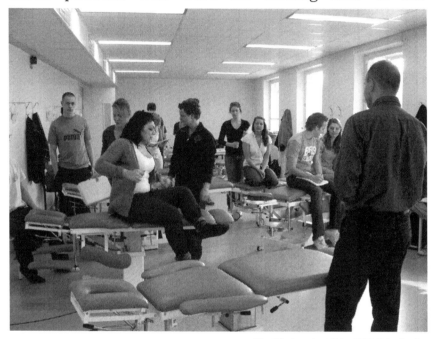

Dr. Kirsten LaVista/SUNM photo

A Naprapathy class in Sweden, where the specialty has become very popular for treatment of musculoskeletal issues.

orthopedists and orthopedic surgeons and given them a course of Naprapathic treatments. Part of the research was to differentiate which patients would benefit from timely manual treatment vs. those that would be better off waiting to see the surgeon. The researchers cited medical literature showing that many general practitioners felt they needed more guidance about where to refer their patients presenting with musculoskeletal issues.

The patients were randomized into a group that would see a Naprapath for manual treatment and a second group that would receive some combination counseling by an orthopedist, medications, steroid injections and pre-surgical diagnostic exams such as x-rays. Over the course of a year, the researchers found less pain and more function among the patients who received Naprapathic treatments, and these patients also perceived themselves farther along on the road to recovery than those in the control group.

In fact, 62 percent of the patients treated with Naprapathy agreed to be taken off the waiting list for surgery, and another 18 percent were found not to need surgical intervention once they had seen the orthopedist.

Another controlled trial in Sweden looking at more than 400 patients with neck and back pain divided them into a group that was treated with Naprapathy, massage and stretching, and a second group in which a primary care physician advised the individual patients how to stay active and cope with the pain. Some patients began feeling improvement within three weeks, the researchers also writing in *Clinical Pain* reported, and significant statistical differences were apparent between the groups at 7- and 12-week follow-ups. Those in the Naprapathy group reported that their pain and level of disability had decreased and many felt they were very much improved from before the treatment.

The conclusion from this trial was that Naprapathy could improve lives for patients when dispensed at the primary care level before it got to the point where they were thinking of surgery.

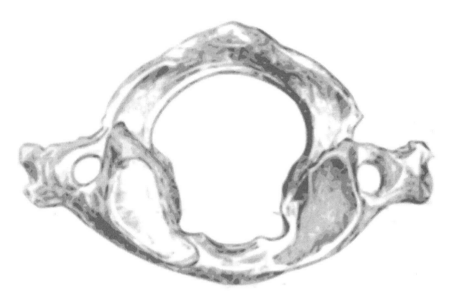

In this illustration of the first cervical vertebra, or "atlas," the large opening in the center is the spinal canal through which travels the spinal cord, the superhighway for nerve communications throughout the body. The smaller openings on each side carry blood vessels and nerve bundles (plexuses) branching off of the spine.

In the U.S., a 2014 survey report looked at military veterans in New Mexico who were suffering musculoskeletal pain from physical injuries and had been diagnosed with PTSD. An important point of this survey was to gauge the psychological effects of Naprapathy treatments along with the physical effects.

As in the Swedish studies, there was a measurable decrease in pain over the course of treatment. Just as importantly among these PTSD sufferers, their psychological status improved markedly. Where most had reported having great trouble sleeping at the beginning of the study, by the 10th week this number was down by two-thirds. Another significant improvement was a decrease in catastrophizing, or feeling that their pain would never get any better. By the 10th week, the patients reported a much lower level of catastrophizing as they physically began to feel their pain going away. This survey proved the potential of Naprapathy in treating PTSD and its associated symptoms.

More recently, the American College of Physicians in 2017 updated its guidelines for the care of patients reporting low back pain based on controlled trials and reviews of non-pharmacological treatment. The new recommendations steered medical doctors to alternative treatments such as exercise, tai chi, yoga, massage applied heat, acupuncture, and spinal manipulation – the last of which, of course, is where the evolution of scientific Naprapathic Manual Medicine began[9].

Patients with musculoskeletal pain often feel that their lives are diminished to the point of despair. One of them was Kathy Simonik, an Illinois woman who had three back surgeries and years of physical therapy, but her pain never went away. Finally, she was referred for an operation that would implant a metal rod in her

---

[9] http://annals.org/aim/fullarticle/2603228/noninvasive-treatments-acute-subacute-chronic-low-back-pain-clinical-practice

back, immobilizing much of her spine. She would never again be able to turn her head. After the failures of the earlier surgeries and looking at the certainty of lifelong disability with the latest recommendation, she sought an alternative treatment, and through a friend discovered Naprapathy.

Profiled in *Prevention Magazine*, Simonik began treatments every two weeks. Gradually, immobility from locked ligaments and adhesions from surgery began to improve, and her pain lessened. She was able to give up her pain medication, and worked with her yoga instructor to where she could do back bends and headstands, which had been impossible for her previously.

Prevention went to an orthopedic surgeon to get his take on her treatment and improvement:

"I tell my patients to try anything and everything before they resort to an operation," said Dr. Noah S. Finkel of Huntington, N.Y. and a spokesperson for the American Academy of Orthopedic Surgeons. "The reason she got better was probably because her therapist (Naprapath) helped break down all the scar tissue she had and stretched out the cramped ligaments around her spine..."[10]

Today, more than 100 years after Oakley Smith had his breakthrough moment, the benefits of his research are helping patients feel better and make more of their lives. Studies continue to show the positive results of Naprapathic treatment, and surgeons understand the mechanism by which it works. Naprapathy has been

[10] Prevention Magazine, September 2007

proven to reduce pain and restore a patient's physical ability. To many people who have suffered and found little or no relief from other therapies, it's the answer they've been looking for.

CHAPTER EIGHT

THE COMPLEMENTARY CONTINUUM

Medicine, from simple and often curious beginnings, has become a broadly diverse and complex body of knowledge and practice. Nobody can know or do it all. Thus, specialties have developed that treat specific conditions, and today's practitioners – very good at knowing what they don't know – always include the mostly unspoken question, "Did this person come to the right place?" in their evaluation of a patient.

TRADITIONAL AND MANUAL MEDICINE:

HOW NAPRAPATHY PLAYS A VITAL ROLE

It's an important, sometimes life-critical, criterion. Healthcare professionals are trained to recognize when a patient is best referred to another specialty for an optimal outcome. Your allergist is not going to perform your heart surgery, and you wouldn't consult a gynecologist to treat your acid reflux. If you present with symptoms that indicate you should go in a different direction for treatment, your practitioner will tell you.

Some may see this as fragmentation, but in reality it is a continuum of care that takes into account the complementary nature of many specialties, and in effect creates a team of multiple practitioners to provide the correct treatment based on their special knowledge and skills.

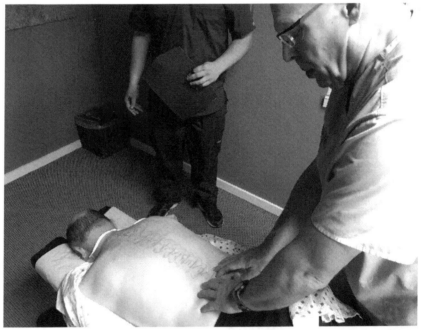

Dr. Kirsten LaVista/SUNM photo

Naprapathic evaluation and treatment at the SouthwestUniversity of Naprapathic Medicine

Musculoskeletal disorders indeed have seen the development of multiple treatment modalities and professional practices. Here is a short primer on who is who, and how multiple practitioners might contribute to your care along with your *Naprapathic Physician*:

We've discussed orthopedic surgeons and the general wisdom that surgery should be a last resort. Sometimes – in cases of major trauma, setting broken bones, repairing birth defects and replacing our worn-out parts – they are sometimes the only specialty that applies to your immediate situation.

But after their work is done on the acute problem, a patient's recovery is complemented by specialties such as physical therapy and massage therapy to help restore function and treat pain and immobility following an operation. Naprapathy, with its focus on connective tissue, is a perfect fit into this continuum. Freeing up adhesions, improving blood and lymphatic flow, and stretching out tight tendons and ligaments will frequently assist in recovery and restoration of movement.

Note that Naprapathy can be useful after many surgeries, not just orthopedic. For example, many survivors of breast and other cancers benefit from Naprapathic treatment to help restore lymphatic and vascular flows where the surgery has removed lymph nodes and severed blood vessels.

Orthopedic surgeons can approach their specialty through two different avenues. The first is the more traditional MD degree and its general training; the other begins with a Doctor of Osteopathy (DO) degree, where the musculoskeletal system is the focus. Both then have five years of surgical residency to complete their training.

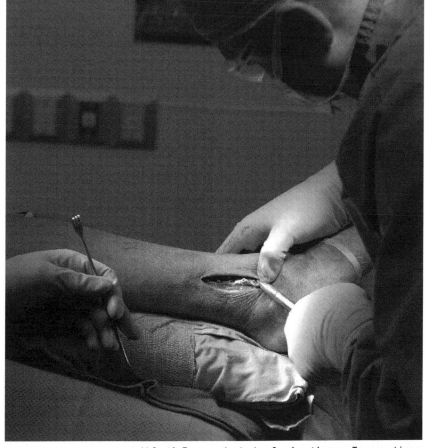

U.S. Air Force photo by Senior Airman Teresa Aber

Air Force Maj. Michael Tompkins, M.D., 633rd Surgical Operations Squadron orthopedic surgeon, makes adjustments to a metal plate in a patient's ankle during a procedure at Langley Air Force Base, Va. Orthopedic complaints are the most common reason patients seek medical care.

The specialists known as *orthopedists* diagnose and treat various musculoskeletal condition, but do not necessarily perform surgery. Osteopaths were the original bone "manipulators," but have largely lost the art of manual medicine practices now performed by Naprapaths and chiropractors as they've focused more on surgery.

Massage therapists are trained to work on soft tissue throughout the body, but do not address any of the spinal issues that we know can cause painful and disabling effects in other places of the body. For example, a massage therapist may work on pain in your

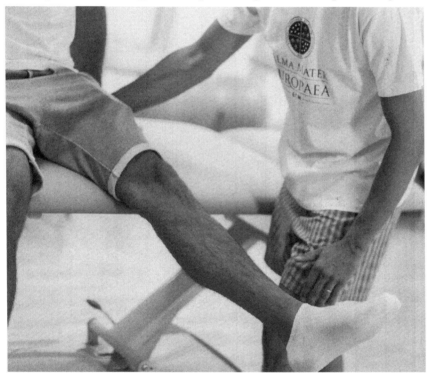

Photo by Free Stajler, licensed under Creative Commons

legs, but would not seek to manipulate the spinal structure, which is likely the fundamental source of the pain.

A *physical therapist* seeks to reduce pain and restore function in specific parts of the body. The treatment they administer in most cases is prescribed by a doctor or another professional who has diagnosed the problem and written a prescription for therapy, such as a podiatrist. Their job is most often seen as rehabilitation for a specific part of the body to achieve a specific goal.

Physical therapy complements many other modalities of treatment, and is very often prescribed after musculoskeletal surgery or injury, and much of their work is focused on strengthening muscles and freeing up connective tissue, though again it does not usually address conditions with a spinal origin. Practitioners of physical therapy are much in demand as the population ages and in recent years are pursuing education and training to the doctoral level, with many of them earning a Doctor of Physical Therapy degree, though it is not a requirement for receiving a PT license.

Both Naprapathic physicians and *chiropractors* need their respective doctoral degrees to practice, and are regulated by the states. As we noted early in this book, Naprapathy developed out of chiropractic more than a century ago, when Dr. Oakley Smith formulated and proved his theory about connective tissue causing nerve and circulation problems, and formulated the treatments that are used today.

Chiropractic treatment is based on high-velocity "adjustments" to the spine to remedy what chiropractors see as displacement, or "subluxations," of the vertebrae. Many people feel better after a chiropractic adjustment, though Naprapathy realizes that such adjustments do nothing to loosen up the connective tissues that are in fact pulling the vertebrae out of alignment. Chiropractic is seen as a temporary fix.

A *Naprapathic Physician* (or *Naprapath*) will like a chiropractor palpate and observe to determine where the spine may be out of alignment, causing leg pain, numbness or tingling in your fingers or any of a myriad of symptoms that indicate a nerve is pinched,

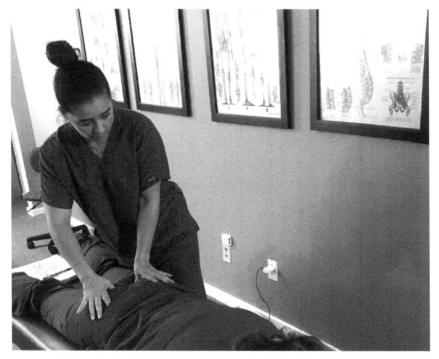

Dr. Kirsten LaVista/SUNM photo

constricted or otherwise unable to do its function. The Naprapath will treat the connective tissue to free up adhesions, scar tissue and other strictures and restore both comfort and function. Naprapathic treatment will not "crack your back" as is said of chiropractic; instead, it will apply vigorous manipulation, stretching and other low velocity manual maneuvers to effect a cure – hopefully long-lasting as is the specialty's intention when treatment begins.

Naprapathy, as noted above, complements other musculoskeletal treatments and specialties. For example, it might be advantageous to combine short-term Naprapathic therapy to free up the fascia and neurovascular bundles and at the same time pursue physical therapy for the rebuilding of the muscles that have been weakened by chronic disability.

There is indeed a continuum of care throughout modern medicine, and especially among the specialties offering musculoskeletal treatment. And among MDs who understand and have access to Naprapathic practitioners, many will recommend that you see a Naprapathic Physician to diagnose and treat a problem that manifests in the connective tissue of the body. For many patients, Naprapathy keeps them out of the surgical suite – and gives them back their lives.

CHAPTER NINE

THE ART OF NAPRAPATHY

The medical establishment through the years has waxed and waned on the value of the physical examination in diagnosis and treatment. Indeed, the ability to diagnose what is troubling a patient has grown more and more dependent on imaging (x-rays, CT scans, ultrasounds) and laboratory processes – which include blood chemistry analyses and the pathologist's microscope – than on the physician's touch. Collectively, this has come to be known as "evidence-based" medicine.

Many medical professionals consequently admit to a "decline in bedside skills" that were once the primary diagnostic vehicle,[11] but in modern practice have in

---

[11] A History of Physical Examination Texts and the Conception of Bedside Diagnosis: Abraham Verghese, M.D., MACP, (*by invitation*) Blake Charlton, B.A., Brooke Cotter, M.D., and John Kugler, M.D. Transactions of the American Clinical and Climatological Association, 2011; 122: 290-311

some ways eroded. Today's medical schools puzzle over how and how much to teach about the physical exam that includes auscultation (listening with a stethoscope), palpation (such as feeling the neck for enlarged lymph nodes and pressing the belly to assess potential conditions such as appendicitis), and visual assessment of the patient.

In Chapter Two we discussed the signs the Naprapathic physician will look for upon first seeing a patient, and the medical history that will be taken to put in perspective the discomfort and symptoms the patient presents with. In manual medicine, the examination will focus on the musculoskeletal system – and especially in disciplines

YOU HAVE TO FEEL IT TO HEAL IT

such as Naprapathy and chiropractic the focus is on the spine and associated structures. A chiropractor is looking primarily for misalignments of the vertebrae ("subluxations"); your Naprapathic Physician will assess not only any spinal issues, but more to the point, how the connective tissues that include tendons, ligaments and fascia have caused and/or contributed to the patient's complaints. The resulting treatment will be based on the results of that examination.

In other words: **You have to feel it to heal it!**

The physical examination by a Naprapathic physician seeks additional information beyond spinal alignment that the doctor can use to decide on how to apply the manual therapy. The muscles in your back might be weak or untoned, or locked in a painful spasm. Nerve irritation may manifest as a tender spot near the spine; tremors or involuntary movements; pain elsewhere in the body such as the leg (sciatica); numbness at the site where the nerve is constricted, or perhaps in another part of the body.

The doctor will manually assess where the problem originates – that is, which bundle or bundles of nerves emerging from the spine may be compromised by the connective tissue that normally would act as a protector. There are 30 bundles in total that are routed from the spinal vertebrae in bilateral pairs to control specific areas of the body, and the examination pinpoints those bundles that need treatment.

Under the microscope in his laboratory, Dr. Oakley Smith discovered that scarring of the connective tissue caused adhesions, immobility and constriction of the nerves, leading to the patient's symptoms. Over more than a century of clinical treatment, his followers have developed and refined the manipulations that will help alleviate those symptoms.

As noted in Theory and Principles of Naprapathy, a paper by Dr. Tony Zayner D.N. and Dr. Kirsten LaVista D.N., "All Naprapathic manipulation is an endeavor to stretch scar tissue," thus freeing up the nerves and restoring their correct function, an outcome acknowledged by Dr. Finkel, the orthopedic surgeon, in Chapter Seven.

The patient will feel their Naprapathic physician move directly from diagnosis to treatment, the goal being to restore function and relieve pain quickly for someone who may have been suffering for a long time. The doctor will apply specific manipulations for each area that is compromised, pushing with low velocity, but with just the right amount of force, to free up the adhesions and constrictions and get the nerve impulses flowing correctly once again.

To you, it may feel like a firm massage, but to the doctor it is a therapeutic movement applied in a predetermined direction to get the scar tissue to give up its hold on the specific bundle of nerves[12] and the accompanying lymph and blood vessels. The doctor may also stretch your muscles and work your joints to help bring back motion where you have been limited. You will feel the tight muscles and connective tissue relax. You are becoming "unglued."

Each manipulation, determined by the physiology of the affected areas of the body and the force and direction needed to break the strong grip of localized scar tissue, is designed to achieve the desired result at the site of the symptoms as well. With sciatica, for example, the Naprapathic physician will work on the area of the back where the sciatic nerve that controls leg movement and sensation emerges from the spine, and then help the patient stretch the tissues of both the back and the legs to facilitate recovery of feeling and motion.

The human musculoskeletal structure is bilateral – that is, the bones, muscles and connective tissue on one side of the body are mirrored on the other. They also serve to counterbalance each other, and when one side suffers an injury, the other side compensates. Think of walking with a sore foot; you will put more stress on the healthy foot than the one that hurts.

---

[12] Theory and Principles of Naprapathy, by Dr. Tony Zayner D.N. and Dr. Kirsten LaVista D.N., Southwest University of Naprapathic Medicine

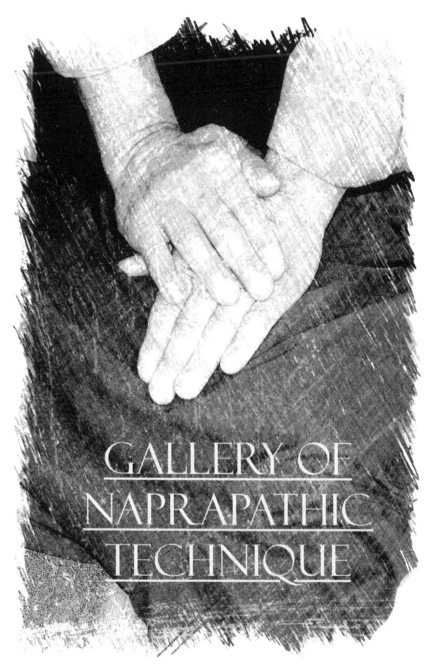

GALLERY OF NAPRAPATHIC TECHNIQUE

PHOTOS BY DR. KIRSTEN LAVISTA

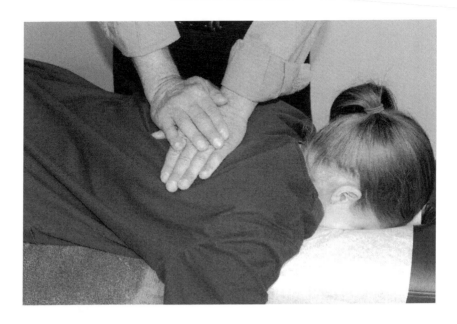

The Double Anteros positions above and below treat the upper back and shoulder blade areas, with different contact points taken by the hands.

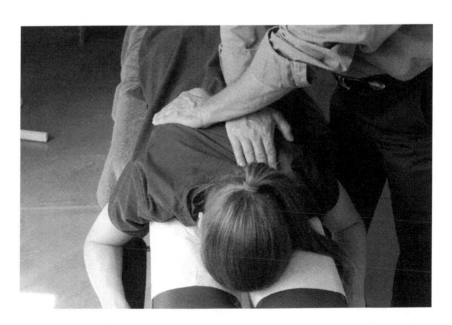

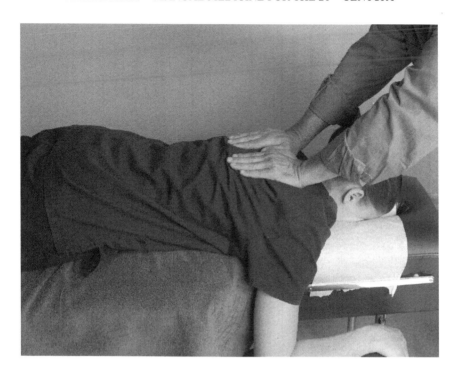

Additional examples of the Double Anteros positions treating the upper back.

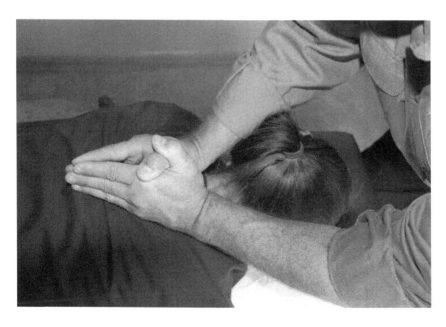

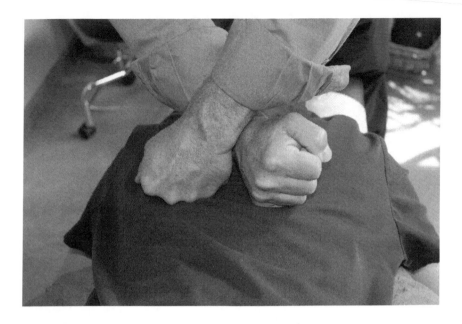

Double 10s above and below treat the soft tissues along the length of the spine. Next page top, Double 11s on the lower spine.

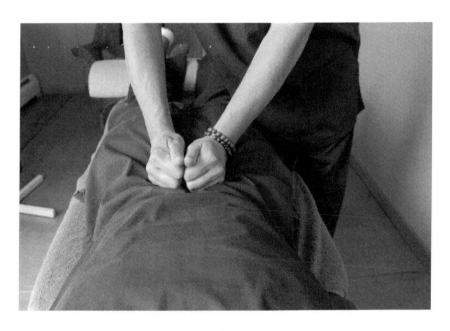

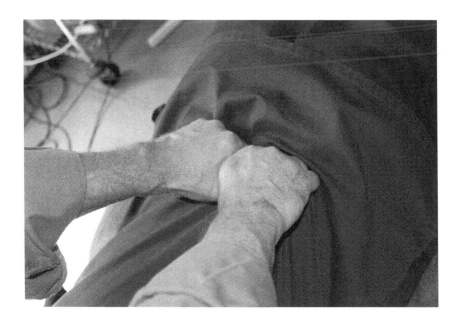

Below, stretching the lateral and posterior longitudinal fibers of the lumber vertebonds.

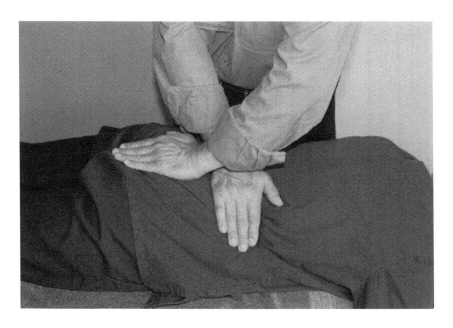

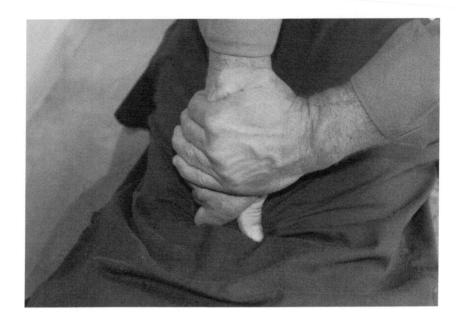

Double Anteros, above, treat the lumbar spine. Below, palpating the area prior to applying the Double Anteros.

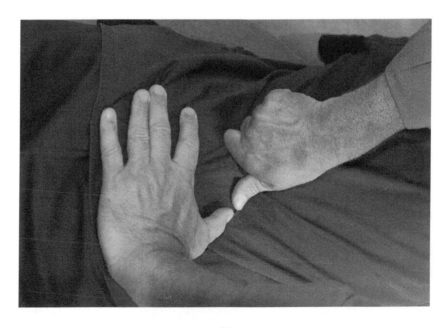

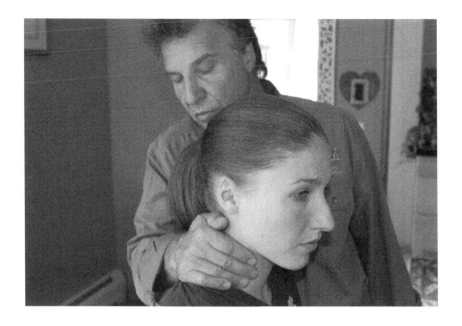

Above, preparation for the Straight Lateral postion on the neck. Below, a Straight Lateral is applied.

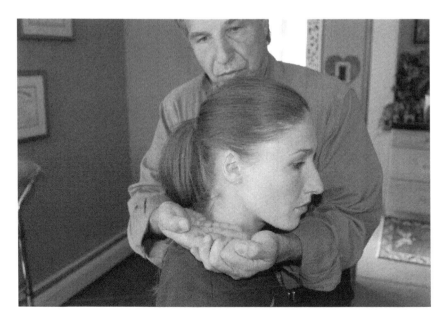

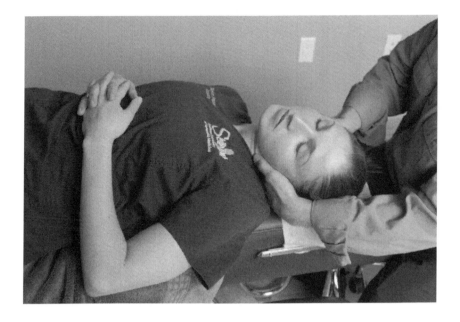

Above, the Straight Lateral is applied with the patient in the supine position. Below is the Postero Lateral.

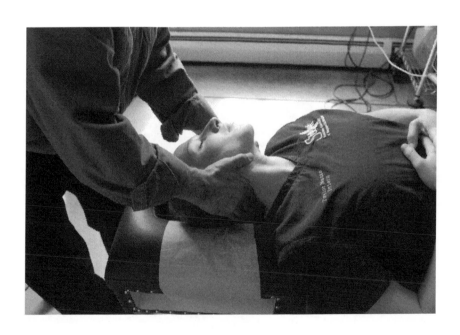

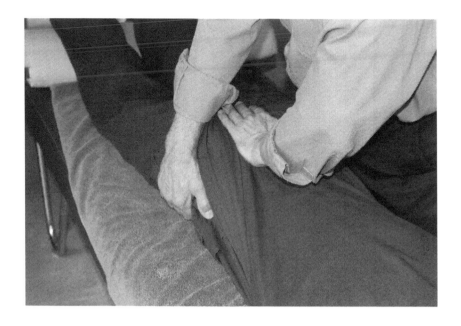

Above and below, stretching the Antero-Posterior fibers of the sacroiliac joint.

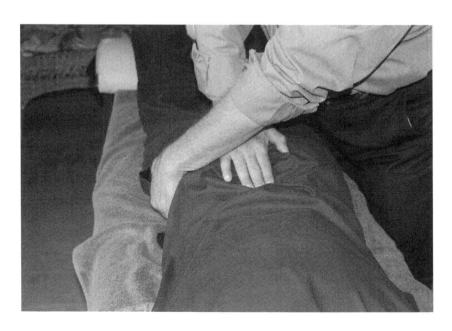

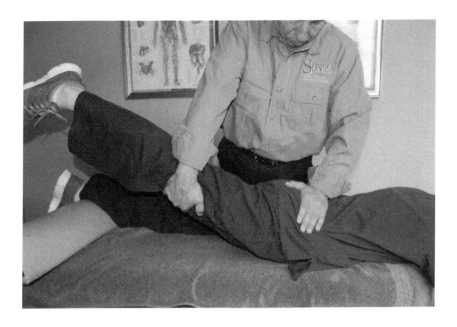

Above, treatment of posterior hip position. Below, Intero Hand, Contact 13 of the posterior aspect of the sacrum.

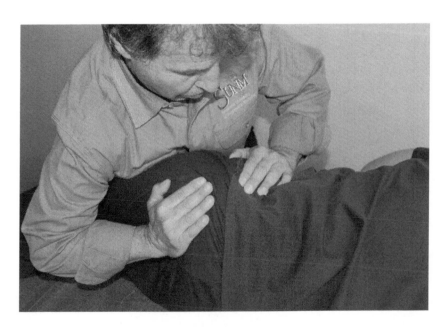

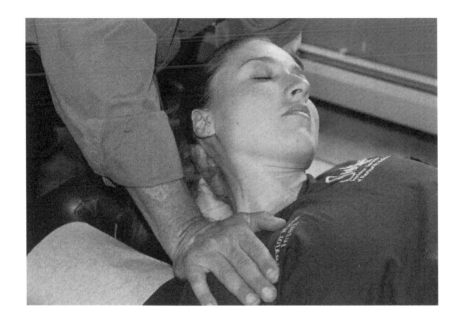

General cervical stretches, above and below.

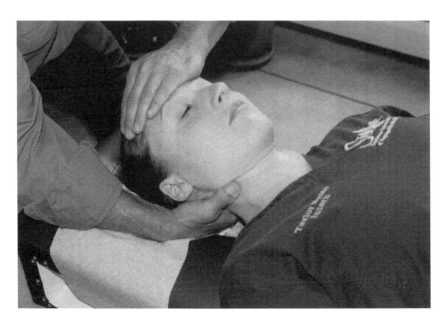

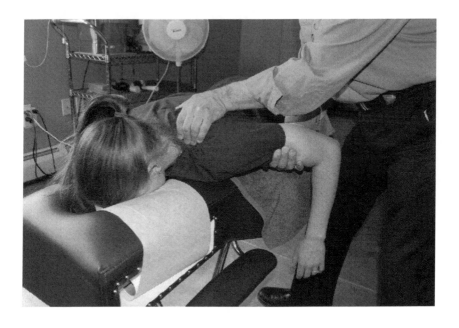

General shoulder stretches.

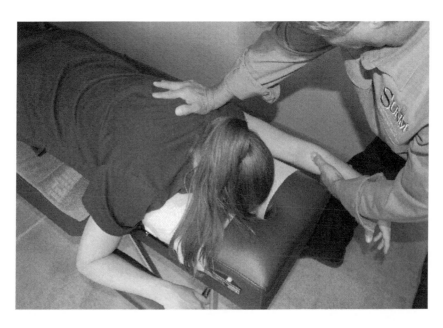

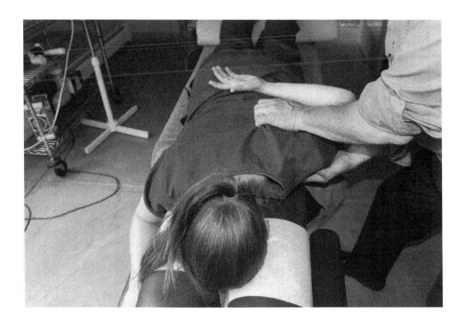

General shoulder stretches, above and an inguinal stretch below.

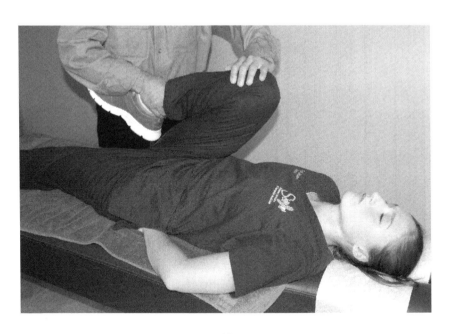

Over the long term, this injury on one side of the body will affect the other, perhaps overstretching the tissues on the left to balance the constricted tissues on the right – and often resulting in pain on both sides.

There is such a thing as "muscle memory," where your body adapts to facilitate frequent actions, like looking in the rear view mirror. Likewise, adapting over the years to an injury on one side of you will pull the other side out of alignment and potentially lead to the constrictions and adhesions that have just been treated by your Naprapathic physician. So, your doctor would likely prescribe certain exercises as continuing rehabilitation to make sure that the tissues continue to stretch and move like they should, and don't fall back into their injured state. The idea is to address the problem and see improvement – as noted before, in just a couple of visits to the office – with active takeaways that will help heal and restore the body over the longer term.

How does Naprapathy differ from other treatment modalities? It is the focus on problems stemming from the soft tissue that distinguishes the practice from others, such as chiropractic. Naprapathy uses low-velocity manipulation to mobilize nerves that have been locked into place and squeezed by surrounding tissue, causing pain and dysfunction. This is based on Oakley Smith's discovery that it is in fact in the soft tissue where the symptoms originate. Chiropractic by contrast uses high-velocity manipulation (which you can often hear as well as feel) to adjust what practitioners perceive as misalignment among the vertebrae, which theoretically puts pressure on the nerve bundles. One reason Naprapathy rejects this approach is that the bones actually provide a lot of room for the nerves to operate freely, since the boney channels through which the bundles run are roughly eight times the diameter of the bundles themselves.

Treatments such as physical therapy and various types of massage therapy also address the soft tissue, but without the laser focus of Naprapathy on mobilizing the connective tissue, and thus the nerves it contains. Naprapathy goes straight to the root of the problem and seeks swift, positive results from treatment.

A Naprapathic treatment may seem quite vigorous, and afterward it may feel like you've had a good workout. The fact is that you have. The doctor is using your own individual anatomy and physiology to work on the scar tissue and adhesions. And while he or she may seem to be doing all the hard work, you are an active participant in the treatment. Just as normal movement involves bone, muscle and connective tissue, Naprapathic Manual Medicine manipulates these structural features of the body to restore normal function and relieve pain. It is a natural treatment based on scientific principles, and offers proven benefits to the patient who may have found little but disappointment elsewhere.

CHAPTER 10

IN NAPRAPATHY PATIENTS' OWN WORDS

N aprapathy is all about making people feel better, treating their musculoskeletal issues in a way that will do the most good. Many patients return to activities they've not enjoyed in years, or return to the workforce to once again feel productive. They avoid surgery and all its attendant risks and lengthy recovery. Naprapathy brings people back to the lives they want and deserve to live.

For Kimberly, an Air Force veteran and mother of two who had suffered musculoskeletal pain and dysfunction since her mid-teens, life had become grim. "I couldn't carry the laundry basket upstairs," she says, "I couldn't pick up my kids. Some days I couldn't stand up straight."

By 2014 she was all but disabled with pain in her rib cage and joints and frequent headaches. Kim was diagnosed with degenerative joint disease and sought treatment from a chiropractor once or twice a week. As a veteran, it was determined she had a 50 percent disability due to joint pains and migraine headaches. Doctors were puzzled over the cause.

"I have been to so many different specialists," Kim says. "They were talking about fibromyalgia, Hashimoto's Disease and other diagnoses." But they couldn't tell her definitively what was wrong, and nothing they recommended really helped. A friend who had heard about Naprapathic Manual Medicine recommended in 2017 that Kim try it.

"It was life changing," she says. After just a few treatments her joint pains and headaches were on their way out. The improvement continued and she began doing things that had been impossible just a few months earlier.

"I feel more limber than I have in three years," Kim says, though she cautions people seeking Naprapathic treatment that the next day they may be sore from the therapeutic stretching and manipulation of their connective tissues. But that goes away quickly, she notes, while the benefits remain.

"I'm getting more sleep. I'm more patient with people. I'm able to get down on the floor and play with my kids," Kim says.

Soon, Kimberly will be moving to Italy with her children and husband, who is still serving in the U.S. military. Kim recounts a recent scouting trip to find a house to rent, and spending up to 18 hours in airplane seats flying there and back, something she could never have done before Naprapathic medicine took away her pain and difficulty moving.

"This is the first time in my life that I feel I am making some real changes and improving my life," she says. "Nothing helped the way Naprapathy did."

Dave Capelli is a retired state police trooper who had been in great shape, as his profession required. But musculoskeletal issues were looming. He was helping a friend with packing and moving when, "I lost the feeling in my right hand."

MDs couldn't find the cause or fix the lack of feeling. Other practitioners were likewise stymied by Dave's symptoms.

"I went to a couple of chiropractors and they told me I had to live with it." It was not the kind of solution that agreed with a person used to taking charge in difficult situations. Dave kept searching for an answer and discovered Naprapathic Manual Medicine.

"Two treatments and the feeling in my arm came back," he relates. It dawned on Dave that other musculoskeletal issues caused by his life of service might also respond to Naprapathy — his knee pain, which doctors had thought might need surgery but which he didn't want, and problems with his shoulders. Soft tissue treatment by a Naprapath continued to work for him.

"Last year I rode over 3,000 miles with my bicycle and motorcycle," he says.

"Many of my friends have had hip surgery, back surgery, their shoulders worked on," says Dave.

"I tell them to get Naprapathy instead."

Rose Armijo had serendipitously come across Naprapathic Manual Medicine in a way that recalls Dr. Oakley Smith's transition from traditional chiropractic.

Pain and limited motion in her back had sent her to seek treatment. "I'm not one to take pills," she says, "but it's so hard when you can't even straighten up."

"I had gone to a chiropractor who very much treated with Naprapathy techniques," working on the soft tissue rather than making that specialty's signature high-velocity adjustments of her patients' joints. The chiropractor, nearing the end of her career, eventually closed her practice, and Rose "went out to find someone who could do the same."

A state government employee with a background in health care, Rose had seen Naprapathy demonstrated in free clinics and workshops for her colleagues. She learned more about Naprapathic practice and agreed with its focus on soft tissue, and appreciated that treatments were based on a detailed plan of care. Along with her back, Rose began to see her Naprapathic Physician for stress that manifested in her neck, as well an old knee injury. Soon her pain was gone.

"It's a modality of care I can recommend," she says. "I know one person who was taking a lot of pain medication. I told her to go for Naprapathy, and now she doesn't have to take the pills."

Manuel Martinez was also reluctant to take pills, but almost fully disabled by fibromyalgia when he was diagnosed at age 45, for a time he felt he had no choice.

"I was in a pretty dark spot," Manuel says. "After that it was steady with constant headaches, pain everywhere, brain fog, all kinds of tests, medications..."

While he avoided the most dangerous opiates such as Oxycontin because of his security clearance and job at a national laboratory, Manuel still needed drugs like the sleep aid Ambien and synthetic opioid Tramadol while he saw countless medical doctors, chiropractors, acupuncturists and physical therapists for relief. But nothing helped.

"I was so exhausted," he says. "Here I was facing disability and I started to think of ways to check out."

His primary doctor encouraged him to leave work and go on disability, but Manuel said "No, I'm not going to go there." Then a work colleague who knew what Manuel was going through suggested he try Naprapathy.

"It helped me. In fact, it saved my life," Manuel says. "People need to try it."

Manuel felt different after his first treatment, and as he continued the pain and dysfunction began to go away. "I started weaning off of the medications," he says.

"You're going to feel it after the first session," he says. And given his condition when he had his first Naprapathy treatment, to feel he was on the road to recovery "did take a few sessions."

Manuel finally felt he "was working toward better health." And today, "I do everything I want to do." Manuel still sees his Naprapathic Physician several times a year, and especially if there's a fibromyalgia flare-up. When he was involved in a traffic accident that left him with a neck injury, he recovered with the help of Naprapathy – and without taking any medications.

Manuel Martinez happily tells people about his experience with Naprapathic Manual Medicine – even handing out his practitioner's cards and information – and has become an advocate for those who also could be helped by it. His primary doctor, after seeing his amazing improvement from near disability, now refers her patients with many musculoskeletal issues to Naprapathic Physicians.

Manuel would also like to see the specialty come to workplace clinics like his at the national lab, where he feels Naprapathy could help everyone from office workers with carpal tunnel syndrome to laborers with muscle strains and back problems. And he'd like to see Naprapathic treatment covered universally by insurance, as his was.

"It would save the system time and money," Manuel says, and he's sure as well that it will save lives of people like himself who are in the "dark place" that Naprapathy lifted him from.

We met Kathy Simonik much earlier in this book. Now it's time to hear a little more of her story. Kathy had been through years of pain and dysfunction, undergone surgeries installing rods in her back, which didn't help, and listened once again as her orthopedic surgeon recommended a procedure that would lock her spine into one ramrod-straight position for the rest of her life.

"I was like a model patient," Kathy relates. "I did everything he wanted me to do." Until, that is, the fateful day when her surgeon recommended the operation that would inalterably affect her life, and she knew it wouldn't be for the better.

Kathy was burdened by her previous surgeries. "When you have metal in there, you feel heavy," she

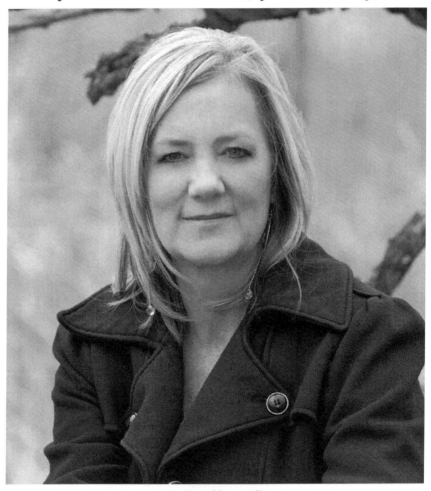

Kathy Simonik

says. Not to mention that the complications of one operation which occurred three weeks after the procedure. One of the screws implanted in her spine broke a lumbar vertebra in half.

Her husband quickly noticed that she was unexpectedly different when they went out for coffee to gather their thoughts after seeing the surgeon. "Why aren't you crying?" He asked Kathy.

"I said, 'I'm not doing it.' The decision was almost easy after listening to everything," she says.

"This time my attitude was different. I thought, 'This is my body. I'm not going that route.' Then I found Dr. Nuzzo."

Kathy came to my office. As she now tells people about our first visit, "He said you're going to become unglued. Everything in me, all the connective tissue, was bound up together."

"He took action."

It was a threshold moment for Kathy. Her orthopedic surgeon had pooh-poohed any mention of alternative medicine, urging her instead to consent to the surgery that would give her even less movement in her back, which already was largely immobile because of the implanted rods. After the new surgery, she would not have been able to turn her neck or twist to the side. Her spine would be locked in place and devoid of its natural curvature. And this would be forever. "I didn't buy his objections," she says.

I began to treat the connective tissues in the area of her lumbar spine — the lower vertebrae that are the location of the pain and dysfunction in many patients. Soon, Kathy says, "I became more fluid in my walking." The pain that she had been taking medication for — and that she Spartan-like tried to hide from others — began to disappear. She was getting her life back without the surgery her doctor had offered and without the drugs.

In an inspired move that would have dumbfounded her surgeon but was so rewarding to me, Kathy decided to open a yoga studio and help others keep their bodies in shape. She now has several studios, and sees customers who are much like she was in the past. "A lot of them come in and they're post-op, and their doctors have just about given up on them," she says.

In fact, her orthopedist had told her not to do yoga; I told her it would be a great idea in between office visits to help loosen up all the connective that had been locked up tight and pulled her body painfully out of alignment. "The doctors had worked to take the curve out of my back," she says. "I had to put it back in."

"I couldn't believe it," when she heard that yoga was something she could and should do, Kathy says. "I still had that block in my head." But as her flexibility grew from the Naprapathic Manual Medicine treatments I gave her, so did her muscle tone and strength. Today, she says, "I can even do a headstand and a handstand."

When I see a patient return to living like Kathy did, I want to do a handstand myself; maybe even turn cartwheels. Helping and healing are the reasons I became a Naprapathic Physician. And stories like those in this chapter make me so happy that I did.

.

CHAPTER 11

WE'VE BUILT THE MODEL

D
elivering health care to a growing, aging population is expensive everywhere in the world, and especially so in the United States. Health care is not a commodity, and it will not come down in price due to high volumes of users. Rather, the costs will continue to rise as more and more people are brought into the health care system.

However, there are ways to be both more effective in providing care and more considered in spending for that care. Musculoskeletal issues are a prime example of a problem where patients can be helped and costs can be contained without making unnecessary sacrifices in the quality of care. Research shows that many, if not most, sufferers can be helped without overly expensive and questionably effective care, including hospitalizations and surgery, for their musculoskeletal pain and dysfunction. People can return to normal, get back their lives, work, play and enjoy themselves again — if the care they get is appropriate for their problem.

Naprapathic medicine is dedicated to restoring lives that have been diminished by musculoskeletal issues. For more than a century, this specialty has employed research findings and treatment modalities that current medical science is only today coming to recognize. Indeed, the study of anatomy is still a work in progress, with structures such as the newly named Interstitium — the body's head-to-toe fascial system, which has been the focus of Naprapathic treatment from the beginning — finally being seen for what they are and do. Those long-dismissed membranes in our bodies have suddenly become important to practitioners, but they were always important to the patients who would benefit greatly by treating their dysfunction.

What's more, traditional medical practice is now realizing that certain treatments that became standard over the years — opioid painkillers, for example — do more harm than good. And that goes against the very first canon of medicine, to "Do no harm."

In 2017, the journal *Annals of Internal Medicine* published an article from the American College of Physicians entitled "Noninvasive Treatments for Acute, Subacute and Chronic Low Back Pain: A Clinical Practice Guideline[13]," one of a growing number of recent treatises to evaluate the effectiveness of alternatives to surgery. Its recommendations ratify those of other studies: doctors should advise noninvasive treatments that include exercise; manual therapies that may

---

[13] Ann Intern Med. 2017;166(7):514-530. DOI: 10.7326/M16-2367
Published at www.annals.org on 14 February 2017 © 2017
American College of Physicians

encompass manipulation of the spine (which Naprapathy gently accomplishes in a low-velocity manner by working with the soft tissue, rather than the high-velocity chiropractors' thrusts marked by the

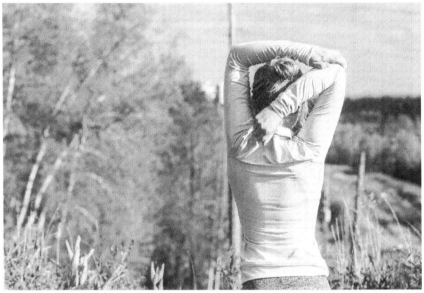

Photo by Jacob Postuma on Unsplash

sound of "cracking" joints), including physical therapy; various massage techniques; yoga and stress reduction; among other conservative treatment modalities.

While Naprapathy was sadly absent from much of the medical literature reviewed in the study, it is interesting to note that some "evidence showed that a combination of spinal manipulation with another active treatment resulted in greater pain relief and improved function at 1, 3, and 12 months compared with the other treatment alone."[14] The key here is to understand that Naprapathy treats our skeletal structure and

---

[14] Ibid.

potential misalignments of joints and bones by freeing up and stretching the connective tissue, relieving tension on the bones and allowing them to return to their correct position.

Additionally, Naprapathic Manual Medicine releases

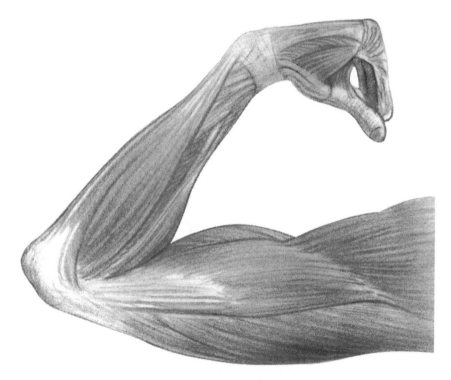

Soft Tissue of the Arm

National Institute of Arthritis and
Musculoskeletal and Skin Diseases
National Institutes of Health

adhesions, strictures and scarring in the fascia that keep the nerve, blood and lymph vessel bundles from passing along signals from the brain and nutrition for our cells, and helps them remove the metabolic waste products such as lactic acid that make us feel tired, sluggish and sore after stressing our muscles. Thus,

Naprapathy, by focusing on the soft connective tissue rather than just the bones and joints, can provide multiple benefits with its unique treatment techniques. Combined with exercise and activities prescribed individually for the patient's particular symptoms, Naprapathic Manual Medicine is a treatment modality that aims to reduce pain and improve function directly and for the long term, not merely mask the discomfort with drugs or limited-duration "band-aid" fixes.

The success of Naprapathy in treating and helping patients has been gaining new visibility on the health care spectrum, and medical doctors who know about the specialty are giving it credit for filling a void in modern treatment of musculoskeletal pain. In a 2009 ABC News story, Dr. Gerard Varlotta, then director of sports rehabilitation at New York University Langone Medical Center's Rusk Institute of Rehabilitation Medicine/Hospital for Joint Disease in New York City, said that Naprapathy "seems to be picking up pieces that other modalities have left behind."

The ABC News story also cited a study published in the *The Clinical Journal of Pain* which reported that patients with back or neck pain given Naprapathic Manual Medicine saw improvement in their symptoms and functionality. Those treated with Naprapathy were 27 percent more likely to experience a decrease in pain, and 18 percent less likely to be disabled than those who were given traditional medical advice and treatment. What's more, patients of Naprapathy were 44 percent more likely to see and feel the improvement in themselves than patients who got only the standard medical therapies.[15]

Currently, Illinois and New Mexico have set the model for Naprapathic care as part of the continuum of modalities used to treat the modern world's all-too pervasive musculoskeletal issues. Both states have

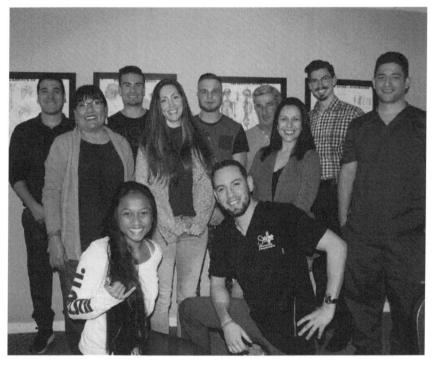

Dr. Kirsten LaVista/SUNM photo

Students and interns at the Southwest University of Naprapathic Medicine

recognized and licensed Naprapathic Physicians, and both have schools teaching the art and science of this much-needed specialty. In these states, Naprapaths' offices are busy seeing everyone from construction

---

[15] https://abcnews.go.com/Health/Healthday/ story?id=6557926&page=1

workers to law enforcement officers, from office assistants to Ph.D.s at national laboratories, and treating them with manual medicine that will often renew their lives. Medical doctors are referring their patients increasingly to Naprapathic Physicians as they see the positive results. And insurance carriers are seeing the benefits of Naprapathy's non-invasive, non-pharmaceutical treatment in helping the members of their health care plans get better at the same time that Naprapathy reduces costs.

Naprapathic treatment is a new direction for many patients to take and for traditional medicine to recommend. But its benefits are becoming clear for all to see, and as the specialty of Naprapathy grows more patients' lives will improve. Indeed, Naprapathic Manual Medicine, after more than a century of practice, is a vital, health-giving solution for so many of the 21st century's health problems.

AUTHORS' NOTE

This book provides an introduction to Naprapathic Manual Medicine and its effectiveness in helping patients who have musculoskeletal pain and dysfunction. However, it is by no means the last word on the subject.

I believe a great future exists for Naprapathy and its treatment of our bodies' soft tissue, helping heal and restore lives that have been diminished by suffering. In our practice it is a tremendous reward to see patients feel better, live better, return fully to their families and work – and return to living their lives.

As a formal discipline, Naprapathy is more than a century old, and as an informal practice it dates back much further. The evidence for its success is established, and I believe that it will contribute strongly to improving health in America, even as it helps relieve the strain on our healthcare system by providing timely, cost-effective care that keeps patients out of the hospital, away from addictive drugs and doing the things they love and need to do.

It is particularly satisfying to see Naprapathic

Manual Medicine blazing a new path to treat age-old conditions. I expect its benefits will become increasingly recognized as medical science continues its discoveries about our bodies and how they work. We have been treating the newly named Interstitium for well over 100 years, but only now has medicine realized that this head-to-toe fascial system is in actuality a functional organ whose own good health is vital for the entire body's well-being.

It leads to many avenues that need to be researched – for example, is fibromyalgia, which Naprapathy is highly effective at treating, indeed a disorder of the Interstitium rather than the ill-defined but crippling syndrome we see in so many otherwise healthy patients.

I am curious, too, about the recent finding by a consortium composed of Harvard Medical School, the Dana Farber Cancer Institute and the University of Vermont that the act of stretching limited tumor size and growth in mice with breast cancer.[16] Researchers speculate that stretching may help the immune system do its job and help keep the cancer at bay.

Again, Naprapathic Manual Medicine would be right on target through its efforts to free up lymph and blood vessels from scarring and constrictions, and facilitate their work in transporting immune system cells to problem areas and carrying away damaged and diseased cells and their byproducts.

Our goal in Naprapathy is whole body health

---

[16] Stretching Reduces Tumor Growth in a Mouse Breast Cancer Model. https://www.ncbi.nlm.nih.gov/pubmed/29777149

through treating the soft tissues that are everywhere in our bodies, and traditional medicine is only now realizing just how important those tissues are. There is much left to be discovered and accomplished, and it's hard to speculate on what our next book on Naprapathy will include. A lot of surprises, I believe, and a lot of hope.

Dr. Patrick Nuzzo, D.N.
Dr. Kirsten LaVista, D.N.

APPENDIX

SUNM Veterans Study 2013

1 February 2013

SUNM Preliminary Survey on Veterans jointly affected by Musculoskeletal Pain and PTSD

BENEFITS OF NAPRAPATHIC MEDICINE ON VETERANS' HEALTH

prepared by Dominique Alò, (Scientific Consultant for SUNM, Southwest University of Naprapathic Medicine—The Lofts 3600 Cerrillos Road, Suite 734 Santa Fe, NM 87507)

| 2 | SUNM Preliminary Survey on Veterans jointly affected by Musculoskeletal Pain and PTSD |

Introductory note:

The aim of this proposal is to seek collaboration between the New Mexico

Department of Veterans Services (NMDVS) and local naprapathic practitioners to

study and implement the benefits of naprapathic medicine in treating veterans

who are suffering from pain as a result of physical injuries and Post Traumatic

Stress Disorder (PTSD). This document will be presented to the appropriate

legislative committee and also forwarded to the New Mexico Congressional

Delegation to seek cooperation and funding opportunities to treat veterans

diagnosed with both musculoskeletal problems and PTSD.

Results from our future analyses will be promptly reported to the above-cited

authorities and will be published in technical reports and peer-reviewed

journals for publication.

| SUNM Preliminary Survey on Veterans jointly affected by Musculoskeletal Pain and PTSD | 3 |

INDEX

4 SUNM Preliminary Survey on Veterans jointly affected by Musculoskeletal Pain and PTSD

ABSTRACT

In this preliminary study we seek to define the effects of Naprapathic treatments on war veterans suffering jointly from musculoskeletal pain and post-traumatic stress disorder. We report the pilot results on a small cohort of veteran patients that show the initial beneficial effects of Naprapathy as an alternative medicine method to treat post-traumatic discomfort and pain. With this initial study we hope to establish collaborations and funding opportunities with governmental agencies. Our goal is to continue the treatment of war veterans affected by joint, musculoskeletal pain, and PTSD, as well as to alleviate their pain at the physical and psychological level.

INTRODUCTION

Health-related problems on veterans of war are a growing concern due to an increasing awareness of the possible long-term consequences of their deployment. Illnesses and symptoms are most often associated with fatigue, muscle and joint pain, headaches, difficulty in achieving concentration, memory loss, sleep disturbances, and skin problems (Kang et al. 2003). Often, the symptoms cited above result in diagnosis of post-traumatic stress disorder (PTSD), which has often been considered a possible long-term consequence linked to war deployment. PTSD falls within a psychiatric diagnostic category, and it is characterized by the development of symptoms following a life-threatening experience that exposed the individual with fear, helplessness, or horror. Therefore, PTSD can be considered a psychological trauma that falls outside the range of usual human experiences. Certain events such as wartime combat or incarceration as a prisoner of war typically lead to more pronounced and longer lasting PTSD symptoms. Research has shown that the prevalence of PTSD among injured survivors of stressful events is higher than that of survivors without physical injury, thus suggesting that secondary stressors (such as severe uncontrolled pain, acute anxiety, future uncertainties, and loss of control) may play an important role in the formation of PTSD (Schreiber & Galai-Gat 1993; Brunet et al. 2007; Thompson et al. 2006). Therefore, physical traumas suffered during combat may be strongly related to the onset of PTSD in war veterans. Treatments aiming to heal or reduce physical inabilities or musculoskeletal pain may contribute significant benefits to the holistic state of mind of veterans. In fact, beside physical improvements, veterans may also experience a relief in PTSD symptoms.

123

NAPRAPATHIC TREATMENTS FOR VETERANS

Complementary and alternative medicine (CAM) includes different kinds of practices, including herbal remedies, yoga, and acupuncture and continues to grow at the international level. Smith and colleagues (2007) reported that approximately one third of US Navy and Marine Corps have utilized some form of CAM. Chiropractic treatments are nowadays considered the primary CAM practice and have been used to treat veterans in the US at a growing pace (Green et al. 2009).

Naprapathic medicine has been practiced for over 100 years to treat pain, and this form of alternative therapy combines manual techniques such as manipulations of connective tissue with physical exercises, stretching, treatment of myofascial tissue, and joint mobilizations (Lilje et al. 2010) bringing spinal alignment without the implementation of forceful techniques routinely used by chiropractors, and providing relief without the use of drugs as in western medicine. Naprapathy constitutes today a large part of the Swedish health and medical care system and it is also common in Norway and Finland. Naprapathy is also emerging swiftly in the United States, as part of a more integrative health science treatment not based on traditional medicine.

The New Mexico (NM) veteran population is 172,595 (2012 VA Data) and since the U.S. administration decided to reduce the size of the Army starting in 2012 from a post-9/11 peak in 2010 of about 570,000 soldiers to 490,000 soldiers by the end of 2017 (Feickert 2013), the expected population of veterans in NM is supposed to increase in the near future. Many NM veterans are already seeking CAM treatments based on naprapathic medicine after their physician's recommendation. Therefore, New Mexico should prepare for these returning soldiers and establish valuable treatment opportunities for those dealing with muscular, skeletal, and joint injuries.

SUNM has already assisted several patients in the last few months and implemented a pilot study to begin treating war veterans affected by both musculoskeletal pain and PTSD. To record our results we developed a comprehensive survey and recorded the data of each physical examination to include several measures for recording the patients' health status across the time period for which they were treated. We report our preliminary results therein, and although this data is only based on a few patients and a limited amount of time, it suggests that most of the patients have already received some beneficial effects from Naprapathic treatments.

OBJECTIVES OF SURVEY

Determine the effectiveness of Naprapathic treatment interventions on armed forces' retirees. The main purpose of the initial therapy was to determine whether naprapathic manipulations on musculoskeletal and joint pain could alleviate discomfort in war veterans diagnosed with PTSD. Furthermore, this study also attempted to determine to what extent PTSD symptoms can be alleviated in veterans treated with Naprapathic manipulations.

QUESTIONS ADDRESSED:

1. Does Naprapathic medicine provide statistically relevant benefits and or relief to war veteran patients?

2. Do Naprapathic interventions on armed forces' retirees improve their pain intensity, pain quality scores, and functional disability levels?

3. Do Naprapathic treatments provide relief to the patient's perception of

    quality of life as it relates to PTSD?

METHODS

For this preliminary study, we monitored US military active duty retirees

diagnosed with service related PTSD (above 50%) across a 10 week treatment

period. We administered 10 Naprapathic treatments over the course of 10

weeks. Treatments started in August 2013 and ended in January 2014.

We treated a total of nine patients (4 females, 5 males), aged between 32 and 68.

Seven of the patients had an ongoing compensation related to their current pain

condition and the rest were thinking about applying to compensation benefits.

All patients were affected from chronic pain condition (with duration of pain

over 4 years). Each patient's visit was accompanied by a systematic pain

assessment and other questions as described in table 1. Complete surveys were

administered at three different time points: 1 (beginning of treatment), 5, and 10

(last treatment). At treatments 5 and 10 we also administered additional

questions to evaluate pain relief and satisfaction of the Naprapathic treatments.

Three SUNM Naprapathic therapy students helped administer the survey and

entered each patient's responses in the spreadsheet for future analysis.

We used a pain assessment tool that integrated the currently

recommended pain assessment domains for clinical trials methodology and

included questions on coping and catastrophizing, health-related quality of life,

economic impact of the pain condition, social security status, and any ongoing

litigation or compensation process. During consultations, the survey recorded

patient's ratings of improvement, or worsening, and the patient's global impression of change scale. The following table (Table 1) lists the questions

posed by the questionnaire for assessment of pain by their typology.

Domain	Instruments for measurement
Patient's characteristics	Demographics, Employment, Insurance 12 questions (Q)
Pain	Body chart and three Numerical Rating Scale (NRS) pain intensity at worst, least, and average.
Coping/catastrophizing	Two Q
Health-related quality of life	Eight Qs
Duration of Pain Condition	Two Q
Physical functions	10 Qs
Emotional functions	Five Qs
Three more pain-related Qs	Duration of pain condition
Economic impact	Economic impact of pain condition
Compensation	Ongoing compensation process?
Patient rating of improvement and satisfaction with treatment	Three Qs in follow-up (5 and 10) questionnaire
Military and PTSD related questions	Seven Qs
Existing/previous medical conditions	27 options
Smoking habits	7 Qs
Health and Nutritional habits	10 Qs

Table 1. Question domains of questionnaire as it was administered to our patients. For the detailed listing of questions please refer to the annexed complete survey and physical exam.

RESULTS:

Herein we report our preliminary results on the analysis and

interpretation of the initial surveys, since we recently completed the recording of

the outcome of the first group of patients (10 weeks treatments). The main

objective was to assess whether war veterans diagnosed with PTSD can obtain

pain relief and to estimate the extent of the latter. We also wished to evaluate the

1 0	SUNM Preliminary Survey on Veterans jointly affected by Musculoskeletal Pain and PTSD

presence of any quality of life benefits from the naprapathic manipulations to which the veteran patients have been submitted during this first trial period. Does perception of pain increase, decrease, or stay stable before and after treatments? Table 2 and Figure 1 show the records related to the patient's perception of worst pain experienced over the course of the previous week. Pain intensity was rated by each patient by placing a mark on a horizontally positioned line with the extremes labeled "least possible pain" and "worst possible pain". As the average numerical pain rating score (NPRS) suggests (Fig. 1), pain or its perception has overall reduced over the course of the 10-week treatments.

Subject	Baseline	Week 2	Week 3	Week 4	Week 5	Week 6	Week 7	Week 8	Week 9	End of Study Status
1	7	5	4	4	4	4	4	4	4	5
2	7	6	4							
3	7	6	5	6	6	7	7	7	7	7
4	10	9								
5	10	8	9	9	9		9	8	8	8
6	7	6	7	4	7	5	4	3	7	4
7	0	3	3	3	1	3	3	4	4	2
8	5.5	6	5	5	5	4	5	4	5	6
9	5	6	3	2	2	7	7	6	5	2

Table 1. "Worst" PAIN INTENSITY (measured in 0-10 NPRS scale, Numerical Pain Rating Scale). Scored on an 11-point numerical scale (0= no pain and 10= worst pain). Blank cells indicate that the patient discontinued treatments (subjects 2 and 4).

| SUNM Preliminary Survey on Veterans jointly affected by Musculoskeletal Pain and | 1 |
| PTSD | 1 |

We also report sleeping patterns across the 10 week study as they show that the

patients' resting habits may benefit from Naprapathic treatments as stated by

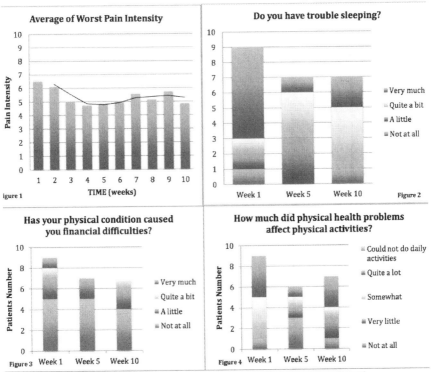

Figure 2, 3 and 4. Health related quality of life. Questions related to sleeping patterns financial status and physical activity limitations. These questions were asked at the beginning of the trial (week 1), in the middle (week 5) and at the end of the treatment (week 10).

each patient. See results in Figure 2 which suggest a slight decrease in "very

much" when patients were asked if the had trouble sleeping. We also report the

results of some other questions related to the patient's perception on their

quality of life. In particular, picture 3 and 4 illustrate the data collected on

| 1 | SUNM Preliminary Survey on Veterans jointly affected by Musculoskeletal Pain and |
| 2 | PTSD |

questions related to the patients' feeling that their chronic pain may influence

their financial status and physical limitations.

The catastrophizing histogram depicted in figure 5 shows data stemming from

the following question: "When I feel pain it's terrible and I feel it's never going to

get any better"; responses show a decreasing trend in the perception of

devastation that can accompany physical pain associated with PTSD.

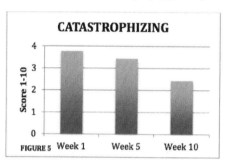

Table 2 shows pain relief as reported by each subject after five weeks of

treatments and at the end of the study, corresponding to 10 weeks. Overall, the

pattern shows that all patients felt some degree of pain relief ranging from 10%

to 90%. Considering that all patients had initially reported having chronic pain,

these results are very promising. Average satisfaction from Naprapathic

treatments shows a positive trend as well and results are reported in figure 6.

Subject	Week 5	End of Study Status
1	30%	10%
3	35%	90%
5	10%	30%
6	50%	65%
7	80%	60%
8	40%	55%
9	80%	85%

Table 2. Pain relief perception as reported by each patient that completed our preliminary study.

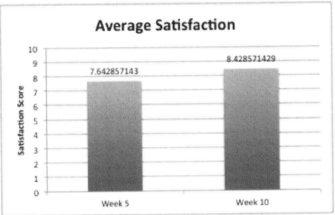

Figure 6. Average satisfaction values measured with a 0-10 scale are reported over each bar.

CONCLUSIONS

We have briefly reported a few significant points emerging from our preliminary results. Although we need some precaution to draw conclusions on data extrapolated from just a few patients and a limited amount of time, we could suggests that our veteran patients have already received some beneficial effects from the Naprapathic treatments over the course of 10 weeks. We hope that results from this initial survey will stimulate more interest in Naprapathic therapy as a very effective CAM treatment for our returning war veterans; as we also wish to improve and extend our study cohort with more funding and collaborations with the appropriate governmental agencies.

AKNOWLEDGEMENTS

We wish to thank SUNM student assistant therapists Julie Grace, Renee Nix, and Taylor Nuzzo for their diligent work with each patient collecting and recording the data. We are also grateful to all the veteran patients that gave us permission to carry out these assessments.

| 1 | SUNM Preliminary Survey on Veterans Jointly affected by Musculoskeletal Pain and |
| 4 | PTSD |

REFERENCES:

Brunet, A., Akerib, V. & Birmes, P., 2007. Don't throw out the baby with the bathwater (PTSD is not overdiagnosed). *Canadian journal of psychiatry. Revue canadienne de psychiatrie*, 52(8), pp.501–2; discussion 503. Available at: http://www.ncbi.nlm.nih.gov/pubmed/17955912.

Feickert, A., 2013. Army drawdown and restructuring: background and issues for Congress. Available at: http://oai.dtic.mil/oai/oai?verb=getRecord&metadataPrefix=html&identifi er=ADA568719 [Accessed April 4, 2013].

Green, B.N. et al., 2009. Chiropractic practice in military and veterans health care: The state of the literature. *The Journal of the Canadian Chiropractic Association*, 53(3), pp.194–204. Available at: http://www.pubmedcentral.nih.gov/articlerender.fcgi?artid=2732257&tool =pmcentrez&rendertype=abstract.

Kang, H. et al., 2003. Post-Traumatic stress disorder and chronic fatigue syndrome-like illness among gulf war veterans: a population-based survey of 30,000 veterans. *American Journal of ...*, 157(2), pp.1–8. Available at: http://onlinelibrary.wiley.com/doi/10.1002/cbdv.200490137/abstract [Accessed April 2, 2013].

Kaptchuk, T. & Eisenberg, D., 1998. CHIROPRACTIC ORIGINs, controversies, and contributions. *Archives of Internal Medicine*, pp.1–23. Available at: http://archinte.ama-assn.org/cgi/reprint/158/20/2215.pdf [Accessed April 4, 2013].

Lilje, S. et al., 2010. Naprapathic manual therapy or conventional orthopedic care for outpatients on orthopedic waiting lists?: A pragmatic randomized controlled trial. *The Clinical journal of pain*, 26(7), pp.602–10. Available at: http://www.ncbi.nlm.nih.gov/pubmed/20639734.

Schreiber, S. & Galai-Gat, T., 1993. Uncontrolled pain following physical injury as the core-trauma in post-traumatic stress disorder. *Pain*, 54(1), pp.107–110.

Smith, T. et al., 2007. Complementary and alternative medicine use among US Navy and Marine Corps personnel. BMC. *BMC Complement Altern Med*, 7(16).

Thompson, W.W., Gottesman, I.I. & Zalewski, C., 2006. Reconciling disparate prevalence rates of PTSD in large samples of US male Vietnam veterans and their controls. *BMC psychiatry*, 6, p.19. Available at: http://www.pubmedcentral.nih.gov/articlerender.fcgi?artid=1476696&tool =pmcentrez&rendertype=abstract [Accessed March 26, 2013].

ABOUT THE AUTHORS

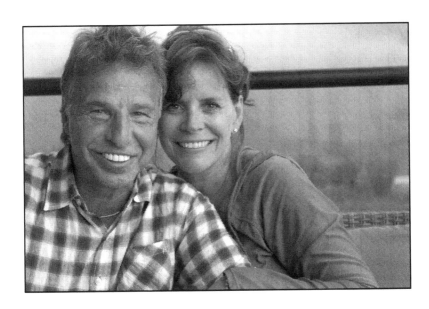

Dr. Kirsten LaVista, D.N. has been a Naprapath since 2000. She was born in Huntington, N.Y. and raised in Arlington Heights, Ill. Kirsten graduated from Prospect High School and Arizona State University, then worked in sales and at an orthopedic clinic while going to Chicago National College of Naprapathy (CNCN).

After becoming a doctor of Naprapathy, Dr. LaVista introduced her new skill to several corporations in Chicago and the surrounding area. She met Patrick Nuzzo in 2003 and moved to New Mexico in 2004, where she co-founded Naprapathic Medicine of New Mexico (NMNM) in 2004, had a beautiful baby boy in 2007, married Patrick in 2009, and co-founded Southwest University of Naprapathic Medicine (SUNM) in 2010.

Dr. Patrick Nuzzo, D.N., has been a Naprapath since 1983. He was born and raised in Chicago. After graduating from Chicago National College of Naprapathy he moved to Escondido, Calif. to work with Dr. Bernard Jensen, D.C. at his Hidden Valley Health Retreat. In 1986 he worked with NFL great Walter Payton and developed sports drinks, bars and antiviral/energy tablets known as RPMs.

Dr. Nuzzo then moved to Santa Barbara, Calif. and started UP TIME sports nutrition. He also worked with Patricia Bragg and Bragg Health products in Santa Barbara.

Moving back to Lake Zurich, Ill., Dr. Nuzzo opened Safe Waters Naprapathic Healthcare. In 1999 he opened a wilderness retreat outside of Silver City, N.M. In 2000, he introduced the Naprapathic Practice Act into the New Mexico Legislature. The bill was passed four years later in 2004, allowing Naprapaths the right to practice Naprapathic Manual Medicine in New Mexico. NMNM was founded in the same year, followed in 2010 by SUNM to train new generations of doctors in the specialty of Naprapathy.

What they're saying about
Dr. Patrick Nuzzo and *Naprapathy, Manual Medicine for the 21st Century*:

Naprapathy stands out as an old and distinct school of manual medicine that holds great promise to address a number of our most persistent health problems. Unfortunately this practice is not well known, but with this timely book, *Naprapathy – Manual Medicine for the 21st Century*, that gap in knowledge is being addressed.

Drs. Nuzzo and LaVista, accomplished Naprapathic practitioners and educators, have succeeded in writing a much-needed text that lifts the veil on this discipline. The text offers a well written and accessible account of Naprapathy that will be of interest to lay readers, policy makers and health professionals alike.

Besides offering a detailed accounting of what Naprapathy is and the modalities it employs, *Naprapathy – Manual Medicine for the 21st Century* makes a compelling case for its increased utilization to address the complex problems of pain management that so heavily burden our health delivery system. Naprapathy in particular offers a practical, cost-effective avenue to provide pain relief in a non-pharmaceutical manner and is particularly relevant in the face of our opioid epidemic.

In conjunction with allopathic medical interventions, Naprapathic medicine holds promise as a therapy which could support a framework of integrative, patient-centric care. Nuzzo and LaVista make a compelling case for expanding the presence of this school of manual medicine and weaving it more directly into the fabric of American medicine.

– John D. Blum, Beazley Professor of Health Law & Policy, Loyola University Chicago

I have been telling everyone I know about the tremendous value of manual medicine ever since I used Naprapathy to help me through the physiological and emotional pain of overcoming a twenty-plus year, four-pack-a-day, cigarette habit. I was fortunate to have Patrick Nuzzo during that most difficult time.

I continued to use Dr. Nuzzo to help me with other ailments, including a painful case of whiplash due to a harrowing car accident. I had suffered whiplash twenty years earlier and was not looking forward to the long and arduous healing process. I was amazed at how quickly I was able to get back to normal activities pain-free due to Napaprathy, which is not only healing, but feels better than any massage I ever had at a fancy spa.

As co-founder of the self-esteem and empathy-building bullying, suicide and substance abuse nonprofit Hey U.G.L.Y., I am sadly aware of how the opioid epidemic is killing many of our youth. I pray this book will open the eyes of parents, the medical community and students who may not know of this holistic healing modality. Opioids are a well-known pain-numbing addiction for youth and adults who do not have the tools to know how to deal with the emotional and mental pain of bullying, stress and that voice in their heads saying they are not good enough, which wreaks havoc on their bodies and psyches.

I am hoping the introduction to Naprapathy in this easy-to-read and understand book will help everyone know what I have known for so many years ... there are better ways to heal and get through pain than using addictive pharmaceuticals.

-- Betty Hoeffner, co-founder/CEO of Hey U.G.L.Y. - Unique Gifted Lovable You

I feel blessed that I was able to meet and be treated by Dr. Nuzzo. In July 2017, upon waking from surgery, I was unable to feel my right leg. I was told that my sciatic nerve had been damaged during the operation, which resulted in me having "foot drop."

After seeing dozens of doctors from July 2017 to April 2018 I was left hopeless. I was told that I would never walk again without the assistance of a brace. I was depressed and resigned that I might walk the rest of my life with a brace and hobble quite uncomfortably.

Then I met Dr. Nuzzo on April 22, 2018, and for once I had hope that I could possibly return to my former active self without a brace.

I flew from Cleveland, Ohio to Santa Fe, NM to be treated. After my first week with Dr. Nuzzo and Dr. Kirsten LaVista, I was able to begin driving with my right foot again – my right calf muscle regained some use immediately. I was shocked and surprised – I had been driving with my left foot for over a year even through I had done extensive physical therapy, acupuncture, chiropractic treatment and medical massage prior to his treatment with little change. However, that all changed after my first week of treatments.

I have since had a second week of treatments with Dr. Nuzzo and since that time I have better circulation in my leg and I am able to walk without the brace. I continue to get better every day. I want to say a nice thank you to Dr. Nuzzo for not only giving me my movement back, but also for the gift of giving me hope and encouragement in the time of despair.

– Attorney Tanya L. Haggins

92575720R00084

Made in the USA
San Bernardino, CA
03 November 2018